My Lovely Choice

Intermittent Fasting for Women Over 50. How to
Live a Healthy Life, Feeling Full of Energy

Sarah L. Moore

Table of Contents

Chapter 9: Real Life Stories From Women in Your Shoes

Bonus Chapter: Intermittent Fasting Kickstart

Introduction

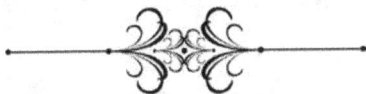

"Youthfulness is about how you live, not when you were born." — Karl Lagerfeld

Disclaimer: The information in this book is not intended to replace the opinion or advice of a medical professional. While significant research has been done and care has been taken to ensure that all of the information presented in this book is accurate and factual, we acknowledge that each individual is different. Should you have specific health concerns that need to be addressed, we always recommend consulting a doctor before commencing with intermittent fasting.

As we cross the threshold of our 50s, women experience conflicting feelings about this period in our lives. If we listen to the hype about menopause and the difficulties we are set to experience, it can be quite a scary prospect to cross that threshold. We cannot deny that there are major physical and emotional changes that come with entering our 50s but these challenges do not have to be insurmountable.

In contrast, our 50s can actually be a time to embrace our femininity as we leave behind a time in our life when we may have had to prioritize everyone else's happiness over our own. From a relationship perspective, we have often settled into a comfortable zone—whether that is within a relationship with a partner or as a strong single woman. We have raised our children and will likely now be watching them flourish, and we are now able to start focusing on ourselves. Our happiness and health is now paramount and it is for this reason, that it is important for us to start looking at options to optimize our health and increase our energy levels.

Some of the health concerns that come with menopause include weight gain and hormonal fluctuations which can cause a wide array of physical issues. As our bodies change, we may find that weight loss methods we used in the past to control our weight, no longer work as well. Most women have that one trusted method of losing weight that works without fail but there is a very good chance that as you move into your 50s, that method will not work anymore. This is likely because, in our 20s and 30s, fad diets tended to do the trick in helping us to shed those extra few pounds but as our body chemistry changes, we really need something more scientifically-based that targets not just calories but the base processes within our body that promote weight loss. Intermittent fasting is one such lifestyle plan.

As women we are told to simply accept that we are going to put on weight as we age but this doesn't have to be the case. All that is required for us to not see ourselves falling into this trap (or dig ourselves out if we're already in it), is a slight mindshift.

The human body is not designed to constantly be fed. Our very original design is actually to eat only when food is available which for our ancient ancestors, was not consistently. Unfortunately, that idea of eating according to food availability has become a problem in the modern age when food is now available on demand. As such, we have also changed our eating patterns so that we are now in a continuously fed state. Our body does not need all of the food we are putting into it and, as a result, it stores this excess as fat. We have been taught that the only way to change this is to reduce the amount we eat and increase our activity levels. While both of those aspects are important to weight loss and maintenance, what is even more important is the time at which we eat and this is where the concept of intermittent fasting comes into play.

The very simple idea behind intermittent fasting is that you allocate a window time of time during the day in which to eat and a separate window in which to fast. There are various protocols that can be followed such as the popular 16:8 protocol, which assigns 16 hours as a fasting window and eight hours as an eating window. This means during your fasting window you eat no food and consume only beverages with no caloric content. During your eating window, you are not restricted unless you are trying to lose weight and then you should try to decrease the number of calories you ordinarily take in.

There are many different ways of fasting. The methods vary in the number of fast hours and days and allowances for calorie where applicable. Intermittent fasting involves abstaining from eating for a set amount of time, before eating normally again. Studies show that this way of eating offers advantages such as fat loss, better health, and increased longevity. Intermittent fasting is easier to maintain than traditional, calorie-controlled diets. Each person's experience of intermittent fasting is individual, and different styles will suit different people.

If you are learning about fasting for the first time, you are likely to be amazed by the range of benefits it offers. There are also additional benefits for women over 50. Some of the benefits you can expect to see from fasting include:

- Weight loss
- Body fat loss
- Decreased levels of insulin
- Increased growth hormone levels
- Activation of autophagy
- Increased energy levels

- Improved mental clarity and emotional stability
- Reduction of inflammation

The range of benefits may make it difficult to believe that this could all possibly come from a single lifestyle change but there is science to back it up. In fact, considering fasting has been practiced for thousands of years, there is also significant social proof of its efficacy. Scientists spend significant time studying fasting because it provides such impactful results.

In a study published in 2014, scientists tested rodent subjects (rodents are predominantly used in such studies due to the extreme process involved in qualifying for human subjects but the results are comparable to human subjects), in fasting conditions and found that intermittent fasting of the subjects protected against diabetes, cancer, neurodegeneration, and heart disease. In non-clinical trials where patients were observed over their fasting journey it was determined that fasting helped to reduce hypertension, obesity, asthma, and rheumatoid arthritis (Longo, 2014).

A very important effect of fasting for women over 50 is the increased levels of the human growth hormone (HGH). As we age, levels of HGH in our body decrease, which means that we find it more difficult to lose weight and we lose muscle mass. Levels of HGH were shown to dramatically increase in the body, which aids in halting, and often reversing, some of the common health conditions seen in women over 50 (Gunnars, 2018).

These are just a few of the benefits of fasting that you can expect to see and the scientific backing behind them. In later chapters, I will go into greater detail and further explain exactly how fasting benefits the body and mind.

My Lovely Choice is a culmination of a lifetime of focus on health and nutrition for me, Sarah L. Moore. I am 55 years old and a dietician and lifestyle coach with a private practice in my hometown of Portland, Oregon. I studied dietetics and biomedicine at the University of Westminster, London. I travel the world with my workshops entitled, *My Lovely Choices.* I am a married mother of two and although I had always wanted another child, I, unfortunately, experienced early menopause at the age of 43 after undergoing chemotherapy for breast cancer. Approximately five percent of women will experience early menopause, which usually starts at around 55 year of age. Although I had built my life on teaching others about the importance of a good diet, I am ashamed to say that my own diet was often less than optimal. During my battle with breast cancer, I discovered the capacity of a healthy diet to stimulate the body's natural self-defense and self-healing mechanisms. The chemotherapy I underwent had a major impact on my body and within a year I was overweight, had wrinkly skin and experienced chronic fatigue. My emotional state plummeted as I struggled to care for my family, and my self-image was very poor. That is when I decided to give intermittent fasting a try. I had used intermittent fasting in the nutritional therapy I prescribed for my clients and I had seen great results in my patients but, for some reason, I had never tried it myself. After experiencing a dramatic change in my own life as a result of commencing an intermittent fasting lifestyle, I decided to start the *My Lovely Choices* coaching business to help share these benefits with other women over 50. I couldn't bring myself to watch other women over 50 struggling with the difficulties of menopause and chronic illness anymore when I knew that there was a relatively easy way to improve their lives. I really felt it was my responsibility to help other women to live their best lives, just as I am now doing. As an independent author, I rely on my readers to share their experiences of my books with others in order to encourage them to read and enjoy the content too. Once you have completed My Lovely Choice and start seeing the benefits of your intermittent fasting journey, please consider availing others to its value by reviewing the book on Amazon **or sign up at the newsletter located at athenapublications.com/**

To be updated on new arrivals and other promotions

As a woman, aging does not have to be scary or uncomfortable. We do not need to be victims of the changes that are happening in our bodies. We are absolutely capable of taking back control and the easiest and most flexible way to do that is with intermittent fasting. As you go through this book, chapter by chapter, be sure to really take in the concepts that are being presented to you.

Understanding how your body works is extremely important for us to be strong, independent women. We need to know how to make our menopause work for us through intermittent fasting, and in order to do that we really need to understand the intricacies of how these processes work. It is my intention, with this book, to prepare you for a lifestyle of intermittent fasting so that you will be armed with the knowledge you need to achieve your goals and enjoy your golden age of life.

Chapter 1:
Intermittent Fasting 101

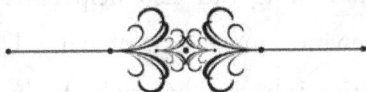

As an age-old practice, fasting has a significant amount of research and social proof to provide a basis for the benefits it claims to provide. When used in the intermittent fasting form, it is possibly the simplest and most flexible regime for weight loss as well the most beneficial for women over the age of 50. Seldom do we find regimes that provide scientific proof of their efficacy in a very specific age group, as well as overall benefits for *all* age groups. Intermittent fasting is one such regime.

Intermittent fasting is an eating pattern that is rapidly increasing in popularity. It involves alternating cycles of 'fasting' and 'eating' windows. Taking in all of your calories within a specific period has been shown to offer a wide array of health benefits. These include weight loss, sustained blood sugar levels, and improved heart health. Fasting can also help enhance mental health and rewind some effects of aging. Unlike many fad diets, fasting is backed by a solid body of scientific evidence. This makes intermittent fasting a healthy weight loss tool with high efficacy rates.

What Is Intermittent Fasting?

The basis of intermittent is that you cycle between windows of eating and windows of fasting. The times for these windows are set by you and can also be structured by choosing a specific intermittent fasting protocol such as 16:8. In this option, you will fast for 16 hours and have an eating window lasting eight hours. We will delve deeper into the various other structures later in the book but suffice to say, intermittent fasting allows for freedom of choice. You are not bound to choose a specific protocol and you can set up your fasting and eating windows to suit your lifestyle. Once you understand the nature of fasting, you will be able to set up your own schedule with confidence.

Intermittent fasting is possibly the only regime, wherein weight loss is one of the benefits, that does *not* dictate what you should and shouldn't eat. When you are fasting, you are only allowed to ingest beverages with zero caloric content such as water, plain coffee or tea. When you are in your eating window, though, you can really eat whatever you like. This freedom, however, should be viewed in conjunction with the understanding that intermittent fasting is not a ticket to binge on junk or processed foods. If you are specifically fasting in order to lose weight, then you will want to try to limit your calorie intake but you needn't do so drastically. The overall rule is to maintain a healthy diet and good nutrition. Plenty of fresh fruits and vegetables, lean protein, and unsaturated fats are all important components of a healthy diet and should be eaten whether you are fasting or not. You may want to slightly change your diet to include foods which keep you feeling fuller for longer as this helps to maintain a steady blood sugar level and reduces the activity of the hunger hormone. By eating low glycaemic content foods during your eating window, you will find it easier to make it through your fasting period.

The Origins of Fasting

The first mention of fasting in historical writing was in the 5th century BCE by the Greek father of medicine, Hippocrates. In his writings, Hippocrates recorded that he had used abstinence from food to assist his patients with specific illnesses. The concept was reinforced, by the fact that physicians noticed that when their patients were ill with specific conditions, they lost their appetite. The physicians saw this as the body's natural instinct to fast while sick. While it would be many centuries before the true science behind this instinct and its benefit during illness would be understood, even in these very early beginnings of medicine, it was understood that food is often not the solution to many maladies. Fasting has long been linked to spiritual and religious practices with many different religions and cultures using specific days of the year to fast in order to cleanse themselves spiritually and mentally.

The concept of fasting became far more sophisticated in the 19th and 20th centuries, as clinical studies began to be carried out on both animals and humans (Rogers, n.d.).

Fasting throughout history has been seen in religious and political instances and today we associate it mostly with the Muslim faith whose followers fast for the month of Ramadan. Each day during the fast of Ramadan, followers begin their fast at dawn and end it at sunset. During this time Muslims are asked to remember those who are less fortunate than themselves as well as bringing them closer to God. Non obligatory fasts are two days a week as well as the middle of the month, as recommended by the Prophet Muhammad.

Although fasting at Ramadan is obligatory, exceptions are made for persons in particular circumstances:

- Prepubescent children are not required to fast although some parents will encourage children to start fasting as soon as they have an awareness of the concept so that they can start to get used to fasting.

- Those who are experiencing illnesses that result in unintentional vomiting are not required to fast.

- Those who are suffering from serious illness are not forced to fast but when the person has recovered they are expected to make up the missed days

- If someone is traveling but one must make up any days missed upon arriving at their destination.

- A woman during her menstrual period is not required to fast, but she must count the days she missed and make them up later.

- A woman who has given birth, miscarried or is breastfeeding is not required to fast for forty days afterwards but she must record the number of days she missed and donate an amount of food equal to what she consumed to the poor

- An ill person or old person who is not physically able to fast. They should donate the amount of a normal person's diet for each day missed if they are financially capable.

- A mentally ill person who may not understand the concept of a fast.

- For elders who will not be able to fast, a lunch meal (or an equivalent amount of money) is to be donated to the poor or needy for each day of missed fasting.

Other religious groups that practice fasting include the Bahá'í faith, Christians, Catholics, Anglicans, and Eastern Orthodox faiths. While many of these religions and faith groups have fasting days on their religious calendars, they have been adjusted through the years to the point where only certain, extremely devout members actually still observe fasting days. Perhaps the most famous spiritual connection to fasting in history is to Buddhism. Buddhist monks practice fasting, meditation, and forms of yoga in order to cleanse the mind, body, and soul and to achieve spiritual awareness. While some refer to the political movements in history who went on hunger strikes in the same breath as the concept of fasting, the two are not really synonymous. Fasting is done to improve the body and mind with no intention to damage the body while people in history who have undertaken hunger strikes for political reasons have done so without care for the damage they may do. The two concepts are quite different.

Throughout history, fasting has been used more and more as a form of medicine and in Europe in the 1980s many fasting clinics sprung up which still exist today. At these clinics, patients would book themselves in to undergo very specific fasting schedules and this would be incorporated with other treatments like special diets and cleansing enemas. For some reason the Europeans have always been more open to the idea of fasting as a medical treatment than the likes of the US or UK. Of course in places like Africa where for many decades food was a scarce commodity, fasting has taken much longer to take off as a form of treatment. Interestingly, though even on the African continent, the traditional tribes have ancient texts that describe the use of fasting by traditional healers.

How Does Fasting Work?

In order to understand how intermittent fasting works, we need to understand the three different states that our bodies move through, as relates to the consumption of food. These three states are:

- Fed state
- Postabsorptive state
- Fasting state

When we eat and digest a meal, we are in a fed state. This state lasts for approximately three to five hours. When your body is in this state, it burns only the food that is directly being ingested. When it has used what it needs, the balance is stored as glucose and fat. Your body is unable to burn off any fat stores when you are in a fed state. The period of time that your body stays in a fed state depends on the natural rate of your metabolism.

Once you move past the fed state and you have digested all of your food, you move into the postabsorptive state. During this time, there is no digestion of food happening in the body. In this state, your body begins to burn off all of your glucose stores. This usually happens over a period of eight to 12 hours, again, depending on the size of the meal you ate as well as your own rate of metabolism.

When you enter a fasted state, your body is able to achieve what we are aiming for—it starts to burn off fat stores. Burning off fat helps you to lose weight and achieve a leaner appearance. By introducing your body to this new state, you access a process that you would not by simply reducing your calories intake (Clear, n.d.).

The Science Behind Fasting

Fasting is the darling of the nutritional research community because it is one of the regimes that consistently produces measurable results in trials. There is, therefore, a significant amount of data available that proves the efficacy of fasting and explains exactly how certain benefits are derived.

We have explained exactly how fasting leads to weight loss and achieving a leaner physique but there is something else that happens when your body is in a fasted state that is a significant health benefit, especially for women over 50. The type of fat stores that your body burns when you are fasting are primarily called triglycerides. A high level of these fats in your bloodstream is a risk factor for cardiovascular disease. Women over 50 are already at high-risk for developing cardiovascular disease so the fact that fasting helps to reduce this particular risk factor is highly beneficial. At this point, it is important for us to point out that your body will only start to break down the protein in your muscles after about 72 straight hours of fasting. You, therefore, do not need to worry about losing muscle mass or experiencing muscle wastage due to intermittent fasting.

Another thing that happens when your body burns fat is that it releases acids called ketones into the bloodstream. Ketones play a powerful role in protecting brain cells against degeneration. Such protection offers a reduction in your risk profile for Alzheimer's disease and even epilepsy. This is clearly a very important benefit for women over 50 as degeneration of the brain and related cognitive issues can start to become an issue as we age. Studies have shown that memory can be improved in just six weeks by increasing ketone levels in older adults. The science behind this is that ketones help to increase brain-derived neurotrophic factor (BDNF) levels in the blood. BDNF is a hormone that naturally decreases in its levels with age and is known to strengthen neural connections in the brain and encourage neuroplasticity, which is the process that happens when the brain learns new things and builds new neural pathways. Neuroplasticity is vital to learning and the development of new habits.

Fasting causes our insulin levels to decrease and, in turn, our human growth hormone (HGH) and norepinephrine levels rise. The increase in the latter two hormones assist with weight loss as well as reducing risk factors for certain chronic diseases. HGH is also known to decrease in our body as we age and lower levels of HGH are associated with larger deposits of fatty tissue. This is one of the reasons that women over 50 tend to develop belly fat and find it difficult to get rid of it. Norepinephrine is a neurotransmitter which also contributes to improved metabolism and fat burning capabilities. When insulin levels in our bodies are high, the rate of conversion of glucose to fat increases. The most prevalent chronic illness related to insulin, of course, is type 2 diabetes. Studies have shown that intermittent fasting is capable of preventing and, in some cases, even reversing type 2 diabetes. Women over 50 are at higher risk for developing type 2 diabetes especially if they are also overweight or obese. Another positive result from reducing insulin levels is that our levels of FoxO transcription factors increase. This hormone is known to help regulate and improve metabolism, increase the likelihood of healthy aging and extend longevity.

During the fasting window, our levels of the insulin-like growth factor 1 decreases. This growth factor, when found in high levels, is considered to be a genetic marker for cancer. The unfortunate truth is that a huge number of cancer diagnoses are made in women over 50, so the sooner you start a regime that can help to reduce your risk, the better.

Fasting is also known to help to reset your internal clock, also referred to as your circadian rhythm. Humans are designed to follow a natural light and dark cycle and our eating is intended to follow that same cycle. Modern man has changed this cycle by staying awake long after darkness falls and also continuing to eat during the night. This disruption causes sleeping problems as well as overeating and sluggish metabolism. Fasting can help to correct this cycle, thereby helping to improve quality of sleep and improve regulation of weight. Studies have also shown that by correcting your circadian rhythm, healing is accelerated in the liver and the health of gut bacteria is improved which stimulates your immune system (Kresser, 2019).

Our digestive system uses the most energy so it stands to reason that giving it a rest, will improve your overall energy levels.

There are conflicting views about whether women should approach fasting differently than men. As women have far more complex hormone systems than men do and, as such, changing the way we eat can have an impact on our hormones. For most, and certainly for women over 50, that is a positive impact, but for some women fasting may negatively impact hormone levels initially. The key here, as with any other regime, is to listen to your body and if you feel as though you are experiencing negative hormonal side effects, reduce the number of hours you spend fasting and try not to fast on consecutive days. The majority of women will experience very little hormonal disturbance due to fasting.

Chapter 2:
The Secret of Self-Eating Cells

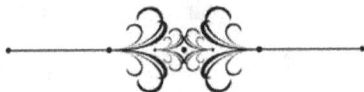

While the phrase 'self-eating' may sound more than a little bizarre, the actual process that we will discuss in this chapter is not so much *Silence of the Lambs* as it is a very normal bodily function. The concept of autophagy was first discovered in the 1980s and it has slowly gained traction in the scientific community. What was once thought to be a process that we had no control over, we now realize is actually entirely controllable and we can, in fact, manipulate it to our own benefit. 'Anti-aging' has become an entire industry and a multi-billion dollar one at that. The irony of this, though, is that the most powerful anti-aging device is free and happening inside your body right now.

What Is Autophagy?

The literal translation of the word 'autophagy,' is 'self-eating'—'auto' means self and 'phagy' means eat. It is a natural process that occurs within our body where cells produce membranes that break down and consume damaged, older, or malformed cells and use the material to make new, healthy cells or for energy. The process is extremely pronounced when we are children but as we age, autophagy naturally slows down. It is this slowing of the autophagy process that causes us to age. Our older, damaged cells are not being replaced with newer and healthier cells at the same rate that they were in our youth. The good news is, that we can use intermittent fasting to speed up the process of autophagy in our body, regardless of our age. Think of autophagy as your body's way of cleaning house. A related process in the body that is linked to autophagy is called apoptosis. This process essentially programs cells to die after a certain number of divisions. It is the dead cells from apoptosis that need to be absorbed and reused.

Autophagy is essentially your body's best anti-aging mechanism. It is the best and most natural way to rebuild your body from the inside out. If we consider that autophagy slows in the presence of high levels of insulin, it is perhaps self-demonstrative that type 2 diabetes is so closely linked with obesity. The higher our insulin levels go, the more difficult it is for our bodies to burn fat and rejuvenate cells (Mangan, 2016). The idea that what we are born with is just what we have to live with is true to a certain extent but with autophagy, time does not have to be against us. We don't have to live in bodies that are basically ticking down to expiration and we certainly don't have to dread getting older because our bodies will 'inevitably' fall apart. There is really no inevitable outcome as we now know that we have a tool that can change all of that. All we have to do is learn how to activate it.

How Do We Kickstart Autophagy?

The autophagy process responds to stress so in order to boost the process we need to put our body under pressure. This has evolved as the trigger for autophagy because it helps us to perform at our peak, even when we are experiencing difficult times. There are three ways that you can trigger and accelerate autophagy in the body:

- Eat fewer carbohydrates
- Intermittent fasting
- Exercise

Reducing our carbohydrate intake can help to accelerate autophagy by forcing our body to burn off fat rather than carbohydrates, simply because the latter is not present. The popular eating plan, The keto diet, is aimed at producing this fat burning state in the body—also called ketosis. The diet recommends that your intake of carbohydrates is limited to five percent of your total food intake. The keto diet is a good way to accelerate autophagy if you do not want to fast. That said, there are several benefits that fasting provides that keto does not.

When we fast, the absence of food in the body alerts the cells to the same type of stress that will trigger autophagy. Keep in mind, that although we consider stress to be a negative thing, in this context it is actually positive. When we refer to stress in a fasting or autophagy context we simply mean that the cells are being put into a more heightened state rather than the sedated state that is experienced when the body is fed.

Exercise is another way that we can put our cells into that stressed state that triggers autophagy. When you work out your muscles experience micro tears that your body is immediately triggered to repair. This repair process includes autophagy. In a study conducted in 2012 on rodent subjects, it was observed that after 30 minutes of running exercise, the subjects were found to have highly active autophagosomes (the membranes and cells related to autophagy). While research is currently being conducted into a chemical stimulant for autophagy, what we know about the negative long-term effects of any chemical introduction into our system makes it quite clear that we are better off focusing on natural methods of triggering the process (English, 2019).

Once we are able to get our bodies into that fat burning state, naturally, we want to keep it there for as long as possible. As you learn about fasting and start to understand how your body responds to the various phases, you will be able to find a "sweet spot" for yourself where you are extending your fast to get the greatest benefit out of autophagy while also ensuring you don't feel ill or uncomfortable. The speed at which you start to boost autophagy will depend on a few factors including your age and physical fitness levels. The fitter you are, the quicker your body will start to accelerate autophagy so it is a good idea to increase your activity levels as much as you can. Exercise does not have to mean grueling runs or endless gym sessions. If you are not very active to begin with, find something that you enjoy to increase your activity levels slowly but surely. Walk the dog more often or jog with friends. Hiking in nature is excellent exercise and emotionally uplifting as well.

Why Is Fasting the Best Trigger?

Fasting is the best trigger to use for autophagy because it is an evolutionary response. Our bodies have evolved to keep us in the best physical condition possible regardless of the availability of food. This is what makes our modern lifestyle so unnatural. We are designed to exist under tremendously difficult circumstances and yet, modern life, most especially in Western countries, has turned us into soft beings that respond only to constant and immediate supply of everything we demand. In the context of our topic, that constant supply is food and we have become convinced that we must eat constantly in order to stay healthy and that is certainly not the case.

While reducing your carbohydrate intake and exercising are both very important things to do in stimulating autophagy, fasting remains the best trigger to use. This is because when we use fasting as a trigger, we don't just stimulate autophagy and then burn the cell matter that is broken down as energy. We also trigger the process of rebuilding healthier, stronger cells in our body. This happens specifically with fasting because of the increase in human growth hormone (HGH), which is a known benefit of fasting.

The process of apoptosis (programmed cell death) can be slowed down and limited by autophagy because, instead of the entire cell dying, autophagy can replace certain components of the cell and rejuvenate it instead. This takes less energy than destroying the entire cell. Apoptosis is the process that causes aging and in reality, eventually death. Cells are only able to survive for a certain amount of time and the cellular structure you are born with is completely different from the one that you have when you are 80 or 90 years old. The link between autophagy and fasting was first discovered when researchers found that if they introduced higher levels of glucagon into a rodent subject, their levels of autophagic activity also increased. Glucagon is the opposite hormone to insulin and, as we know, when we fast insulin levels decrease. Our glucagon levels then experience an equal and opposite reaction and increase. This boosts autophagy.

When autophagy is slow in older people, old, diseased cells begin to accumulate in the body, and disorders can develop. The two best examples of conditions caused by slowed autophagy are Alzheimer's Disease and cancer. Alzheimer's Disease occurs when abnormal proteins build up in the brain. Autophagy can help to reduce this build up by replacing these damaged cells with new cells, thereby slowing degeneration.

It is important to keep in mind that as much as stress on our cells and resulting autophagy is a good thing, as with anything else, moderation is the key. Excessive or continuous autophagy can be damaging to your health. It is for this reason that fasting is not recommended on several consecutive days without a break in between (Jung, 2016).

The concept of autophagy as an aid in preventing chronic disease is a simple one and very easy to understand. It is also quite easy to demonstrate as children, who have a faster natural rate of autophagy, heal from disease and injury much faster than older people. While we may never have put much thought into why this is true, it is, in fact, autophagy that is behind it.

Autophagy and Cancer

Just as autophagy triggered by fasting is beneficial in degenerative brain diseases such as Alzheimer's Disease, it is also beneficial in the reduction of the risk of cancer. Cancer is among the leading causes of death around the globe and it is also a huge risk for women over 50. When autophagy naturally slows with age, the damaged cells build up in our body and can form tumors and other forms of cancer. While the advent of chemotherapy and radiation has gone a long way to helping increase the chances of surviving many cancers, these treatments are still toxic to the body. Nutritional restriction and intermittent fasting are quickly becoming approved methods of cancer treatment when combined with radiation or chemotherapy. Studies have shown that by stimulating autophagy by fasting, the efficacy of traditional treatments is increased (Antunes, 2018).

All cancers begin in the same way. Defective cells form in your body for various reasons and while your body already has processes in place to deal with these cells, as we age, those processes slow down and this is the reason that cancer diagnoses are so pronounced in older people. Of course, we know that it is not only older people who are diagnosed with cancer so this explanation is not a cover-all for every case. Even babies can be diagnosed with cancer and the reason for this is clearly not a build-up over time of damaged cells and there will be other factors at play in such cases. Cancer is an extremely complex disease and if autophagy was the simple solution to all forms of it then we wouldn't still be searching for a cure. Increased autophagy is a preventative measure and gives you a greater chance of not developing cancer as you age. As more is learned about how autophagy impacts the body on a cellular level, we may be able to use it in a further accelerated form to help people with highly advanced forms of cancers and give them a greater opportunity of recovery.

The Major Scientific Contributors to Fasting and Autophagy

One of the major contributors to the field of fasting as a lifestyle is Doctor Valter Longo. Doctor Longo is currently a Professor of Biological and Gerontology Sciences and Director of the Institute of Longevity at the University of Southern California at the Leonard Davis School of Gerontology in Los Angeles which is one of the leading centers for research on aging and age-related disease (Longo, n.d.). Doctor Longo is also the Director of the Longevity and Cancer Program at the IFOM Institute of Molecular Oncology in Milan, Italy (Longo, n.d.).

He studied biochemistry as an undergraduate at the University of North Texas, and received his PhD in Biochemistry from UCLA, where he worked under calorie restriction guru Roy Walford, MD. He completed his postdoctoral training in neurobiology with longevity pioneer, Caleb Finch, PhD. He also received extensive training in immunology, endocrinology, microbiology, genetics, molecular biology, and pathology.

The focus of his studies on the fundamental mechanisms of aging in simple organisms and mice and on how these mechanisms can be translated to humans, directed his interest to the role of fasting. The Longo laboratory has identified some of the key genetic pathways that regulate aging in simple organisms and has shown that the inactivation of such pathways can reduce the incidence or progression of multiple diseases in mice and humans. His laboratory has also developed both dietary and genetic interventions that protect normal cells while sensitizing cancer cells to chemotherapy— interventions now being tested in many US and European hospitals.

The Longo laboratory recently published key findings on a five-day periodic dietary intervention called Fasting Mimicking Diet (FMD), and showed in randomized clinical trials that FMD reduces the risk factors and markers associated with aging and diseases. His most recent studies focus on the use of FMD interventions to activate stem cell- based regeneration to promote longevity.

Doctor Longo's work including his two books has contributed greatly to the concept of fasting being taken seriously in the medical and scientific community. He has constructed very specific diets around the principles of intermittent fasting that focus on the needs of adults in general, breastfeeding women, pregnant women, and children and adolescents. He has also constructed a range of recipes that can be used on this eating plan. These recipes are mainly plant-based foods but also include fish protein sources. Doctor Longo's research in the field of the role of nutrition and fasting is applied to areas such as cancer treatment and he describes the efficacy of his Fast Mimicking Diet (FMD) as a "powerful new weapon" in the fight against cancer. Longo also addresses degenerative brain disease in the application of his theories and much of the research available agrees with his views on this subject.

Amongst others recommendations to avoid degenerative brain disease, Longo suggests incorporating at least 50 milliliters of olive oil and 30 grams of nuts in the diet per day. He also recommends drinking between one and four cups of coffee per day depending on your risk profile. His recommendation to include at least 40 milliliters of coconut in the diet per day is prefaced with the caveat that this is not ideal for those at risk of cardiovascular disease. Coconut oil is, after all, like other tropical oils, a saturated fat. Longo recommends eliminating all animal protein from the diet except for low-mercury fish and all dairy products except for goat's milk. His theories include a high nourishment diet in the fight against degenerative brain disease including as much omega-3, B vitamins and vitamins C, D and E as possible.

With regard to trials Longo conducted related to cardiovascular disease he has found that an FMD showed the following results in participants:

- A reduction in belly fat and circumference
- A major reduction in the inflammatory risk factor protein

- A reduction in total cholesterol and bad cholesterol levels
- A reduction in systolic and diastolic blood pressure
- A reduction in the levels of fasting glucose (Longo, n.d.)

Another major contributor to these fields—but this time in the area of autophagy—is the Japanese cell biologist Yoshinori Ohsumi who won the Nobel prize in medicine in 2016 for his work on cell aging, which includes autophagy. Ohsumi's work determined that fasting activates autophagy and helps to slow down the aging process while having a positive impact on cell renewal. His research has created an entirely new field of science. When Ohsumi started researching autophagy there were only 20 papers published on the subject per year. Now there are more than 5,000 each year as it is such a diverse area of research and one that produces excellent research results (Blue Zones, n.d.).

The research done by giants in the field like Longo and Ohsumi is paving the way for the science behind fasting and autophagy to be centralized as medical treatments. If we are able to get to a place in the world where fasting is actually prescribed by doctors as a treatment, we will see a great equalization in terms of the level of care received by all economic classes as, quite clearly, it costs nothing to implement fasting in our lives. This promise for the future is, perhaps, an even better reason for us to start implementing intermittent fasting as a lifestyle for ourselves right now. If we can get ahead of the curve, we can be part of the social proof that will give these concepts even greater reach across the globe.

Chapter 3:
The IF Golden Age Glow

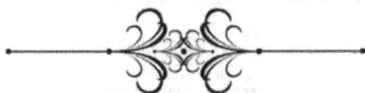

Intermittent fasting provides a wide array of benefits for people of all ages as well as specific benefits for women over the age of 50. One of the most dramatic life changes that is experienced by women over 50 is menopause and it results in some symptoms that can be difficult to manage. Thankfully, there is scientific proof that fasting and autophagy can assist with these symptoms. Too many women struggle with menopausal symptoms in silence believing that it is their lot in life to suffer through menopause. This is not only inaccurate from a medical perspective but it is also an archaic societal idea that needs to be banished. As we work toward equality in our society, perhaps one of the most important struggles is to get these 'old' ideas out of our own head. Women are not forced to handle hormonal difficulties simply because we were born female. Rather, it is our responsibility to ensure that we use all of the tools available to us and change the trajectory of the female story. There is absolutely no need for us to go quietly and meekly off into our 50s and onward and simply accept what is put in our path. Just as nature gives us these challenges as part of our female evolution, it also gives us the solutions to overcoming these obstacles.

Overall Benefits of Fasting

The overall benefits of fasting include:

- weight loss and maintenance
- increased levels of human growth hormone, which naturally declines with age
- increased levels of antioxidants in the bloodstream to limit oxidative damage to cells, which leads to disease
- stabilizes blood pressure
- reduces cholesterol levels by reducing triglycerides in the blood

- fasting gives a break to your digestive system and effectively resets it

- autophagy helps to repair and rejuvenate the body's cell structures

- fasting improves mental clarity and cognitive functioning

- fasting helps to prevent and reverse the effects of chronic diseases including diabetes and heart disease

- practicing intermittent fasting helps to save time as you spend far less time on meal preparation

- resets your circadian clock to get you back into a natural cycle, which is beneficial for digestion and sleep

Specific Benefits for Women Over 50

The major health challenge that women over 50 face is navigating the changes that occur in their body during menopause. While menopause can start from as early as the age of 35 (referred to as early onset menopause), it is most common between the ages of

45 and 55 and is marked by a woman not having menstruated for approximately 12 months consecutively. Menopause is triggered by the natural aging process of the ovaries which causes certain hormones to be excreted in lower quantities. These hormones include progesterone, estrogen, luteinizing hormone (LH), follicle-stimulating hormone (FSH) and testosterone. The follicles in the ovaries also stop releasing eggs for fertilization. Due to the major impact that hormones have on the human body, there are many different and varied symptoms that can be experienced during menopause. Not all women will experience the same symptoms and the severity will also differ from person to person. The symptoms of menopause include:

- weight gain or a difficulty losing weight in certain areas of the body
- vaginal dryness
- insomnia
- anxiety
- depression
- memory problems
- difficulty concentrating

- constipation
- dry skin, mouth and eyes
- reduced sex drive
- headaches
- loss of fullness in breast
- increased body hair growth
- racing heart
- painful breasts
- increased urination and increased occurrence of urinary tract infections
- stiff joints
- thinning out of head hair (Huizen, 2019).

While this list may seem utterly terrifying, it is not intended to frighten you, if you have not yet started menopause. Knowledge is power and if you understand why menopause occurs and what to expect, you are better able to manage your symptoms and avoid having the impact on your life be too severe. Intermittent fasting is an excellent way to limit the impact of menopause on the body.

Menopausal weight gain is possibly one of the biggest problems that women over 50 experience. The reason it is so impactful is that it not only has physical effects but also emotional health effects. When you are overweight, you generally don't feel at your best emotionally and if you suffer from depression and anxiety, being overweight can increase the severity of these conditions. Carrying excessive weight is also linked to the development of many chronic conditions including type 2 diabetes and cardiovascular disease. Any excess weight gained should, therefore, be your first focus during menopause in order to avoid all of those knock-on effects. Thankfully, this is one of the areas where intermittent fasting provides its most powerful benefits (Brusie, 2017).

The most predominant area of concern within weight gain for women over 50 is the fact that belly fat, specifically, becomes very difficult to lose. While before your menopause, you may have seen weight gain in your buttocks and thighs, this shifts during and after menopause to being predominantly focused on the belly area. This belly fat is more dangerous than fat in any other area of the body because it is metabolically-active, which means that it actively releases fatty acids such as triglycerides into the bloodstream. High levels of these fatty acids increase the risk factor for cardiovascular disease in women over the age of 50 (Gillaspy, 2015). From a scientific perspective, in order to change this accumulation of fat, we need to do two things:

- Even out our hormone levels
- Avoid eating in such a way that encourages fat deposits

We have already discussed how intermittent fasting encourages the burning of fat over sugar and it is this process that helps us to lose the menopausal belly fat. So by practicing fasting as a lifestyle, we can help our bodies to get into the fat-burning stage more quickly and more often. The collection of health risks related to belly fat is referred to as metabolic syndrome. Metabolic syndrome is diagnosed when a patient suffers from at least three of the following five conditions and also has belly fat present:

- High blood pressure
- Obesity
- High blood sugar
- High levels of triglycerides in the blood
- Low levels of lipoproteins, which help to rid the body of fat

Avoiding the presence of belly fat or reducing it if you already have it is, therefore, a major contributor to overall good health in women over the age of 50 and this can be achieved through fasting. An interesting link has been made recently, between a lack of vitamin D and the development of metabolic syndrome. Vitamin D is primarily absorbed by our bodies through the skin from sunshine so taking that brisk walk outdoors is seemingly more beneficial than we think.

Fasting is also known to reduce inflammation and oxidative stress, so joint stiffness and lower back pain, which are often more pronounced in women over 50, are eased. Improved bone health has also been observed in certain subjects during studies on the effects of fasting. This is believed to stem from the fact that fasting affects the way that hormones work in respect to bone-essential minerals like calcium and phosphate.

From an emotional health perspective, intermittent fasting may also reduce the effect that depression and anxiety have on women over 50. Even if you have never suffered from either of these disorders before, it is possible for you to develop them, even in mild forms, during menopause. Studies have shown that women who tried various fasting protocols saw an improvement in their mood (Gillaspy, 2020).

The cellular repair process of autophagy and its known acceleration by fasting is another important benefit to consider for women over the age of 50. If we can improve our internal anti-aging system, we are far more likely to develop fewer diseases, see increased longevity and overall better lifestyle quality.

The impact that intermittent fasting and autophagy has on the onset of degenerative brain diseases such as Alzheimer's Disease is also an important factor to consider for women over the age of 50. Added to that is the general cognitive benefit seen from increased autophagy during fasting. One of the most frustrating symptoms of menopause is the memory loss and changes in cognitive functioning that occur due to the changes in hormone levels. This is annoying as well as frightening, especially if your job requires high levels of cognitive functioning. Thankfully, this particular side effect of menopause is usually temporary and balances itself out when your hormones do, but while you wait for that to happen, you can significantly improve the situation through fasting.

As we get older, our own vulnerability starts to become evident and we start to consider that perhaps life is shorter than we thought it was in our 20s. Fasting, when practiced as a lifestyle, has been proven to extend longevity. In a study conducted on rodent subjects, those who were fasted every second day, were found to live 83 percent longer than subjects that didn't (Thrive Naturals, n.d.). So much of what happens in life is out of our hands but our health, for the most part, is within our realm of control. If we use the tools that are available to us we can look forward to an enjoyable "golden age" filled with health and vitality.

Boosting Your Glow

During your fasting window, you should not be taking in anything with a calorie content so water and herbal teas are your best bet. You can improve the taste of these beverages by infusing them with tastes like mint, lemon, lime and cucumber which, also, have no calorie content. Another way to improve the benefit from these fasting beverages, is by using essential oils.

Essential oils have a wide range of benefits on their own but when combined with fasting, you can see exponential results. The following are some essential oils that can be used to aid the body during fasting:

- Cinnamon bark is known to maintain insulin levels, which will help to avoid dips in insulin that make you hungry
- Lavender is an excellent support for the nervous system
- SclarEssence is helpful in maintaining the balance of hormones
- Lemon aids in maintaining the lymphatic system
- Rosemary improves circulation
- Basil and peppermint improve focus and cognitive functioning
- Thyme helps to boost the immune system

You can use these essential oils in herbal tea or infused in water to aid your fast (Warren, 2019).

If you don't want to infuse essential oils into your beverages, you can also get great impact from using them in essential diffusers which you can purchase at any essential oil shop. In a diffuser, rosemary is good for concentration, focus, and clarity. Neroli essential oil has a sedative effect so it is helpful in easing anxiety that may come up as a result of trying a new lifestyle such as fasting.

Intermittent fasting can help to reduce many of the symptoms of menopause and, as such, improve our experience during this time in our lives. By starting with a fasting lifestyle we can also assure ourselves of long-term benefits after menopause.

Chapter 4:
Frequently Asked Fasting Questions

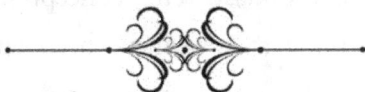

As we gain knowledge about fasting and consider taking it on as a lifestyle, it is important for us to understand all aspects of it. It is also important to ensure that we have all of our questions answered so that we begin this journey with as much certainty and knowledge as possible.

In this chapter we will answer some of the most commonly asked questions about intermittent fasting as a lifestyle, how it might impact you, and we also address the question of who should not be fasting.

What About Breakfast?

The 16:8 protocol of fasting, which we will cover thoroughly a little later in the book, basically means that you are skipping the meal that we would ordinarily call breakfast. This concept seems to go against everything that we have been taught about eating. How many times were you told as a child that breakfast is the meal of the day and most important to our overall health? Food companies, through their marketing have also tried to convince us that if we don't eat a meal in the beginning of the day, something horrific will happen to our bodies. This is simply not true. If you think about the word 'breakfast,' it literally means, to break a fast. If you eat in in the morning when you wake up, the 'fast' that you are breaking is the period during which you were asleep. The origins of this meal, though, were actually intended to break a fast that was longer than that. When the word 'breakfast' was termed, people ate their final meal of the day before sunset, which meant that they really were experiencing a much longer period of not eating than we do now. In fact, when they broke their fast, it wasn't done when they got up. When the term was coined people had many household and homestead duties to attend to before they could even think of eating so they would eat their last meal before sunset, sleep, wake up, attend to their duties and then eat their first meal of the day probably closer to 10 am or 11 am. Is this not exactly what we are suggesting with intermittent fasting?

If you eat a satisfying and nourishing meal the night before, you will actually have more than sufficient energy to get you through to your first meal of the day when fasting. For many people breakfast is enjoyable simply because of the types of foods that are 'prescribed' for breakfast. Cereals, oatmeal, eggs, and toast are all delicious and enjoyable and this idea is among the reasons that people balk at the thought of missing breakfast. You aren't missing breakfast, though, you are simply delaying your first meal of the day and when you do eat that meal, you can eat whatever you want including your favorite breakfast meals. If you really feel that you cannot do without a meal in the morning then you can structure your fast differently and stop eating earlier in the day. It really is up to you as there are few strict rules when it comes to fasting.

What About Eating Every Three Hours?

There was a time in the development of the theory of nutritional sciences when we were told (as scientists believed it to be true) that eating a small meal every three hours was the best way to improve your metabolism and avoid gaining weight. The science of nutrition has moved on since then but, unfortunately, this idea has stayed stuck in the minds of many. It was thought that if we ate smaller meals more often, then we could constantly keep our bodies in a state where it was burning fuel and therefore never create fat deposits. What we now know, though, is that it does not help us to continuously burn sugar. If we eat more than we burn, no matter how often we eat, our bodies will eventually start to deposit fat. Eating more often does nothing to improve our metabolism, all it really does is force our body to stay in a constantly fed state and use huge amounts of energy in our digestive systems. As you learn to challenge your existing beliefs about nutrition and food consumption in general, keep in mind that we are fed data as it is discovered and confirmed by researchers but we are also provided with the data that mainstream media chooses to release. Studies about nutrition and eating plans are published within medical communities and unless a mainstream media publication decides to latch on to that research and make it public knowledge, you will only likely find out about new developments when it is too late for you to put them to good effect in your own life. This is why it is vital for us to question and do our own research through academic resources. It is also important to consult medical practitioners as they are privy to new developments and research that the general public is not aware of. Information that we were given about the best way to eat was certainly correct in its time and there's no conspiracy to keep updated information from you, but if you don't ask, you will never know. If we don't replace old, outdated ideas with newer and more advanced concepts, we are doing ourselves a disservice. There is also a twist to this release of knowledge in that it is sometimes in the best interests of corporate food marketing companies for us not to be aware of updated research and data as this may change our buying patterns.

What About Starvation Mode?

As we have mentioned in other parts of this book already, fasting does not put you into starvation mode, in fact, you are going to have to try very hard to ever really see true starvation mode and you should not want to go there either. What fasting does is it puts you into the very healthy stage before starvation mode in which you are burning your fat reserves. You will only start to run out of these fat reserves after about 72 continuous hours of fasting.

One of the biggest obstacles we face in accepting the idea that we can continue on for several hours in a row without eating is our own mindset. We have been conditioned by food companies and the like to believe that we have to take advantage of the continuous supply of food that is available to us. The truth, though, is that this never-ending fed state is killing us as a society. It is turning us into an entire generation of overweight and ill people who obsess about food. Fasting can help you to change that (Clear, n.d.).

The muscle loss that is seen in starvation mode (as well as some calorie restricted diets) does not occur in fasting because the natural process is burning your fat first. Fasting is actually a great way to become lean without losing any muscle mass. One of the main reasons that people balk at the idea of choosing not to eat for certain periods is because much of the last few decades have been spent on a campaign to raise awareness about true starvation and under nutrition in poorer countries across the globe. That image of a starving child has stuck in our heads just as the campaigns intended it to. The irony, though, is that undernutrition is no longer the world's worst nutritional crisis, it is now actually overnutrition. We have still held onto the belief that we should eat all of our food because there are starving children in the world, though, and so we do, and we feel strange considering the concept of not allowing ourselves to eat whenever we want. After all, shouldn't we be grateful that we have access to food? Why would we want to deny ourselves? This is where we need to change our mindset as we aren't 'denying' ourselves, in fact, we are 'allowing' ourselves. By choosing intermittent fasting, we are giving our body permission to eat only when it needs food and to return to its natural state, which is the opposite of the constantly fed state that we are now in. It is all a mindset change, just as most major lifestyle shifts are and if we can make the change to the way we think, then the physical aspect is far easier.

Can I Exercise While Fasting?

You can exercise while fasting and you should because it helps to increase fat burning. Depending on your individual body, you may find it difficult to exercise during your fasting window and, in that case, you can eat a small snack to break your fast in the beginning of your eating window and then exercise during your eating window instead. Increased physical activity brings a load of additional benefits to the fasting regime so, where you can easily increase your activity levels, it is highly recommended. In chapter 8, we will explore exercising while practicing intermittent fasting more closely.

What Side Effects Can I Expect?

In the beginning of your fasting journey, you may experience some side effects. The severity of these side effects will differ from person to person. These side effects will ease naturally as your body adjusts to its new eating routine. Side effects of fasting can include:

- memory fog
- constipation
- headaches

- light-headedness
- difficulty sleeping

The most predominant side effect of fasting is hunger.

How Can I Deal With My Hunger?

When you get started with your fasting journey, you may find it difficult to adjust to the feeling of hunger. You can be assured that this will eventually level out and your body is simply adjusting to a better pattern of eating. Use the beverages that you are allowed to consume during your fasting window to help you stave off hunger. Consume water and herbal teas with no additives when you feel that hunger is becoming difficult to manage. Your level of hunger will also depend on the type of meal you eat before you start fasting. Try to select foods that have a low glycaemic index (low GI) so that your insulin levels remain constant. Sudden dips in insulin levels can activate the release of the hunger hormone ghrelin which will increase your feeling of hunger. Predominantly, the hunger response is mental and you can think yourself into and out of hunger more easily than you realize. When you feel hungry and you are not sure if you can make it through your fasting window, remind yourself why you are doing this. You are not punishing yourself or forcing yourself to do anything. You have made a choice to fast because you want to give yourself the gift of the whole package of benefits that come along with it. Remind yourself that hunger is temporary but the long-term benefits that you will receive will last a lifetime.

The good news is that your hunger will get easier to manage as your body gets into a new routine of eating. With every successful fast, you will also become emotionally and mentally stronger and more capable of achieving your fasting goals.

Should I Set Goals for Fasting?

Yes, you should definitely set goals for your fasting journey. If you are wanting to lose weight through fasting, set manageable and realistic goals for yourself with set time periods. The best goals are based on the S.M.A.R.T. criteria:

- **S**pecific: detailed
- **M**easurable: a method of gauging your progress

- **A**chievable: push yourself but don't punish yourself
- **R**ealistic: take your circumstances into account
- **T**ime-bound: put a date on it

A specific goal is very detailed, in fact, you should include as much detail as possible. For instance, it is not sufficient to say, "I want to lose weight by fasting." Instead, you should specify the exact amount of weight you would like to lose by fasting. It is a good idea to split large goals up into smaller achievable goals so if you have a significant amount of weight to lose, don't set one goal to lose it all at once. Rather, split the amount up into several parts and set separate goals for your progress. This method is easier and provides greater motivation. A measurable goal is one that you can judge your progress by. When setting your goal, ask yourself how you are going to measure your progress, if there is no measurement tool for your progress then you have likely not made your goal specific enough. Achievable goals are ones that you know you are capable of reaching. You did not put on all of the weight that you want to lose overnight so it is not likely that you will lose it in a short space of time either. This links in closely with the realistic component of the SMART goal. Fooling yourself is not going to help anyone. Be kind to yourself and face the reality of your situation. If your home life or job does not allow for fasting during certain hours, be honest with yourself around that and set your goals to match your reality. The time-bound component of goal setting is perhaps one of the most important. It is not helpful to set a goal without a due date as you will never know if you have actually achieved your goal or not and it doesn't help you to move ahead with other goals if you don't know when to measure yourself on your current goal. Ensure that you make your time allocation realistic as well.

Health goals outside of weight loss will be a little more difficult to set but you could measure goals like reduction of chronic disease by the severity of your symptoms as well as test readings or how much medication is required to manage your symptoms.

A journal and vision board can be very useful tools in tracking your intermittent fasting journey. You can use a journal to visualize where you want to be when you achieve your goals and to make notes of how you feel at certain times so that you can learn from your experiences. A vision board helps you to see your goals right in front of you every day. Seeing your success before you achieve it can be a powerful steering tool to that achievement. For weight loss, the most powerful visualization is yourself. Try to find a photograph of yourself when you were at the weight that you wish to be. Using pictures of other people is not really useful or emotionally healthy as your goal is to be a better version of yourself, not someone else entirely.

Can My Blood Sugar Go Up During Fasting?

In certain people, the process of your body increasingly burning stored sugars and fats for energy instead of food can cause a spike in blood sugar. This is not necessarily dangerous or anything to worry about as long as it naturally moves back to a normal level and does not stay elevated for an extended period of time.

Can I Still Fast If I Suffer From Low Blood Pressure?

Yes you can although you will need to see a doctor first and follow their advice. The key to fasting with any condition is to ensure that you are listening to your body and taking a break if you need to. If you are prone to feeling light-headed due to your low blood pressure at a specific time of the day, you can consider structuring your fast around that time rather than around your sleep.

Who Should Not Be Fasting?

Anyone who suffers from a chronic condition should consult their doctor before they commence with intermittent fasting. Women who are pregnant, breastfeeding, or trying to conceive should also not start fasting at this time. Anyone who has suffered from an eating disorder in the past should stay away from fasting as well as any other eating plan or regime which involves structuring eating times. People with emotional attachments to food may be triggered by fasting. Children under the age of 18 should not be permitted to undertake intermittent fasting unless instructed to by a doctor.

Fasting is very safe but in order to maximize your chances of success, you will definitely want to pick a time to start that is not particularly stressful (Gunnars, 2018).

Can I Fast If I Have a High-Stress Job?

People who work in high-stress positions such as emergency responders, police officers, firemen, paramedics, and emergency room doctors can definitely still benefit from fasting but they will need to structure their fast so that it does not interfere with their work. Most predominantly, in the beginning of a fasting journey, those first few days are quite difficult and you can experience memory fog and difficulty concentrating. In such a case, it would be preferable to start the fasting journey when you are on vacation so that you give your body time to adjust and become used to the way it works under fasting. Fasting while you are on shift if you do one of these jobs can be quite tricky as, often, you will have to eat when you have time. You can definitely still fast if you have a high-stress job where performance has life and death consequences but you will need to be more careful about how and when you start and when you schedule your fasting windows.

What Can I Eat in My Eating Window?

The short answer to this is you really can eat whatever you want to eat but that does depend on what your goals are. In general, a healthy nutritious diet is best to support your body's functions as well as autophagy. If you intend on losing weight, you may want to restrict your calories but you absolutely have to know what your starting point is before you do this to avoid restricting yourself too severely. Going from a 4000 calories diet to a 2000 calorie diet and adding fasting to that is going to be disastrous. First get your fasting journey going, then you can start thinking about restricting calories. You may be surprised by how much weight you are able to lose without restricting any calories and then you can work from that point. One of the old food ages that really does still apply is, "You are what you eat." The challenges you see in your body on a daily basis are as a direct result of the food you put into it. Even disease, both chronic and occasional is caused by the food you eat to a large extent. If food is such an important part of our beings, why then would we choose to simply shovel any junk into our body? Food should definitely be enjoyed but a large part of what you see as personal preference when it comes to certain foods is actually just a mindset that needs to change. If you have always hated vegetables and you hold onto the claim that you don't like them as an adult because you were force-fed them as a child, ask yourself how true that really is. Have you just told yourself that story so many times that you have made yourself believe it? And if that is the case, who are you really helping by continuing with that narrative? You are certainly not helping yourself.

Is Fasting Dangerous for Women Because of Changing Hormones?

The answer to this is not cut and dry. Fasting does have an impact on hormones but in most cases it is a positive impact. It will also have a different effect for different people because our hormonal set-ups are so unique. For women over the age of 50 this is a very important aspect to understand and, as such, we will expand on it in detail in the next chapter.

Chapter 5:
IF and Hormonal Health—
What You Need to Know

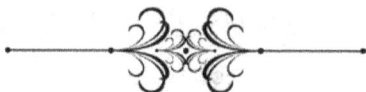

The female body is a complex piece of mastery. We have hormones that operate throughout our lives at different levels to aid in reproduction and all of the processes that go along with it. As much as these hormones are necessary to our bodily functions, when they are out of whack, they can create absolute chaos. Puberty, pregnancy, and menopause are the three periods in a woman's life when hormones are the most likely to be out of their ideal alignment. This can result in side effects across a wide spectrum and it is important for us to understand not just when to naturally expect hormonal changes in our body but how our own behavior and actions can impact our hormones. Menopause can also increase your risk for certain conditions like osteoporosis. You may find that getting through menopause requires little medical attention. Or you may decide you need to discuss symptoms and treatment options with a doctor.

You will find resources that recommend that women avoid fasting entirely. This is not one of those resources. Instead, we will provide you with an understanding of the concepts that you need to make this decision yourself. We are all uniquely built and what works for you may not work for someone else. Many of the giants of medical research who have made fasting and autophagy their life's work recommend fasting for both women and men.

The Low Down on Estrogen

As we age and our ovaries age with us, they signal less frequently for the release of the reproductive hormones. The predominant hormone which, when reduced in levels, signals the onset of menopause, is estrogen. Estrogen plays a role in our bodies throughout our lives. It is responsible for the onset of puberty, controls the thickening of the lining of the uterus during the menstrual cycle, and also ensures that the lining maintains its strength and thickness during pregnancy. Estrogen is responsible for breast growth and changes both in puberty and during pregnancy. It is involved in bone health and the metabolism of cholesterol and plays a role in the signaling of food intake requirements, weight control, the metabolism of glucose, and how sensitive we are to insulin. If you consider these numerous and varied roles, there is no wonder that, during menopause when those levels start to drop, we experience such a wide array of side effects.

In our 40s, we enter a period called perimenopause when we are still producing estrogen in our ovaries but the levels are slowly decreasing. When the production of estrogen has stopped altogether, this is when you are in menopause (Ginta, 2017). During perimenopause, your body is beginning the transition into menopause. That means that hormone production from your ovaries is beginning to decline. You may begin to experience symptoms that we associate with menopause, like night sweats or hot flashes. Your menstrual cycle will not cease during the perimenopause stage, but it may become irregular.

The first signal that you will likely tie in with perimenopause is your menstrual period becoming less regular. As your menopause journey progresses some of the physical changes you can expect to see in your body include breasts losing their fullness, joints becoming stiff, skin and hair becoming dry, lubrication in the vagina is reduced, and fat deposits may start to accumulate around the belly whereas before, you may have experienced weight gain in different areas. The experience of menopause is different for everyone and, as such, so will the symptoms be experienced at different levels and in varying ways by individuals.

Intermittent Fasting and Hormones

The issue of belly fat caused by hormonal changes and how intermittent fasting can help with that, has already been addressed. Another difficulty in menopause is poor quality sleep. This can be caused by hormonal changes causing insomnia or it can be caused by hot flashes making it difficult to sleep. When we don't sleep well our mood, energy levels and even our digestion is affected. Intermittent fasting is able to assist with this by resetting the circadian rhythm and getting us back into our natural light/dark cycle.

Fasting is different for women than for men simply because we have delicate hormonal balances. Some women cannot fast because their hormones become too deeply impacted. This is far more common in women younger than 50, though, because it is impacting their menstrual cycle. For women over 50, this is not an issue but it is always important to listen to your body and make changes where you need to. There are some actions that women can take to avoid any negative impact of fasting on their hormone levels if that becomes a problem. A woman's reproductive hormones (like estrogen) are closely linked to her metabolic function and this is another thing that makes fasting slightly trickier for women than men. When our bodies experience a lack of food, our brain tells us that we need to go into preservation mode so it holds onto energy reserves and increases hunger hormones so that we get the message that food is not present (in case we hadn't already figured that out!). It also then slows down the processes around reproduction because it believes that you need to keep yourself alive and can't maintain a pregnancy too. This would ordinarily not be an issue if those reproductive hormones didn't also impact so many other areas of our body. The trick for women is to convince your body that you are not starving so we don't push our fast into extended periods.

It is recommended that women do not fast on consecutive days. If you fast on Monday, for instance, then only fast again on Wednesday. This gives your hormone levels an opportunity to adjust where necessary. Keep your fasting window to a maximum of 16 hours. We will discuss the different protocols in the next chapter. While many women successfully fast for longer than 16 hours without any negative impact on their hormones, an individual assessment is always required. It is always preferable to start slow and work your way up. Some sources recommend not including intensive cardio exercise on the days that you fast. Again, this is a personal choice and you should listen to your body. If you do find it too difficult to include heavier exercise on your fasting days, you can stick to a walk, yoga, or Pilates (Kanehl, n.d.). If you are in perimenopause and still experiencing occasional menstrual periods, it is not recommended to fast when you are experiencing a period.

Signs to watch out for are extremely low energy levels and intense cravings for very specific foods. A craving for red meat for instance may indicate that you are low on iron and a craving for citrus fruits could mean that you need extra vitamin C. It is also important to keep an eye on your hydration levels because becoming dehydrated can mimic the symptoms of low energy and make your fast much more difficult.

Health Traps to Avoid Over 50

Hormones become a big focus for us as we enter our 50s and we can make the mistake of putting too much emphasis on them and forgetting other issues that are just as important.

One of the major mistakes women over 50 make is prioritizing reproductive health over heart health. We are so often told to look out for the signs of breast, ovarian, and uterine cancers that we overlook our heart health as being another important area to focus on.

The reason that women over 50 are more frequently diagnosed with cardiovascular issues doesn't have to do with hormonal changes during menopause. Rather it is during this time that we see an accumulation of our bad habits from the past coming back to bite us. Smoking, poor nutrition habits, and low activity levels cannot be maintained forever without us seeing the negative impact somewhere along the line. We also see changes in our body during menopause which, when added to our other risk factors, significantly increase our chances of being diagnosed with a heart health condition. It is important to note that although a family history of heart disease will increase your chances of developing the condition, you cannot base your risk profile solely on whether your mother suffered from heart disease or not. Thankfully, all is not lost if you have just hit 50 and suddenly realized that you may now be paying for a lifetime of poor health habits. Any positive change that you make at any stage of your life will contribute toward better heart health. It is never too late. Stopping smoking would be the biggest single contributor to improved heart health. A study conducted in Germany among a mixed group of women and men aged between 50 to

74, showed that within five years of giving up smoking, their risk factor for cardiovascular disease decreased by 40 percent. It is also important to keep up with your cholesterol, blood pressure, and blood glucose screenings. In addition to these, there will be additional screenings that your doctor will recommend, after the age of 50, such as bone density tests. These tests are very important to carry out and you should avoid falling into the trap of skipping them because you don't feel they are necessary. The following is a list of vital screenings and test that are required after the age of 50:

- Colorectal cancer screening
- Pap test and pelvic exam
- Breast exam and mammogram
- Skin check
- Dental checkups
- Eye exams

Another common mistake we make as we head over the 50 mark is believing that the side effects of menopause are inevitable and something that we have to suffer through. There are many methods of treating and reducing the impact of menopausal symptoms.

We have discussed how fasting can assist with this and there are other methods that can be used as well. Urinary tract issues can also be addressed by seeing a doctor and with a wide variety of medications, devices, and exercises. The side effect of menopause that you have the most control over is the emotional aspect. While you may find this time frightening, it is important to remind yourself that you are not the powerless victim of a process that you have no control over. There are actions that you can take and precautions which can be taken to improve your experience of menopause (Raymond, 2015).

Hot flashes can also be very disruptive but another practice just as ancient as fasting is showing excellent results in helping women over the age of 50 to deal with this menopausal side effect—meditation. Hot flashes and, while sleeping, night sweats, can be annoying and embarrassing but when they are severe, they can impact quality of life quite dramatically. Until recently, most women who sought treatment for hot flashes only had hormone replacement therapy (HRT) as an option. This, unfortunately does not work for everyone and it can also increase the risk of certain cancers and heart disease in some women.

Alternative therapies such as meditation and cognitive behavioral therapy are now being recommended as an option more often and with great success. In a study conducted with a group of menopausal women over four weeks, the group was guided in meditation activities which they initially did under instruction and then on their own. Overall, the subjects noted a decrease in hot flashes by up to 40 percent. This study seems to suggest that much of the experience of hot flashes and night sweats is aggravated by anxiety and as meditation helps to reduce anxiety and maintain focus, this makes all the difference to the woman's experience of the symptom rather than the actual physical occurrence of them (WebMD, n.d.).

Common Chronic Diseases in Women Over 50

It is vital for us to remain aware of the risk factors of the chronic diseases that are common as we age. Our age, of course, is not necessarily the determining factor but it is the accumulation of poor lifestyle habits that result in these chronic conditions becoming prevalent at this age.

Cardiovascular Disease

This is an umbrella term used to describe a wide array of disorders which result when a blood vessel that supplies the heart with oxygenated blood becomes narrowed or blocked and also includes any condition that may cause heart muscle damage.

There are some risk factors for cardiovascular disease that are out of the realm of our control. These include aging and having a family history of the diagnosis of cardiovascular disease. The majority of risk factors that contribute to heart problems, however, are within our control. These controllable factors include hypertension (high blood pressure), smoking, high levels of bad cholesterol, a lack of physical activity, excess weight, and type-2 diabetes. If you have many of the unavoidable factors, then it is very important that you eliminate any of the risk factors that are within your control. Risk factor grouping has been proven to hugely increase death rates due to heart conditions or cardiovascular disease. Women with two major risk factors, for instance, have a death rate from cardiovascular disease three times higher than women with only one risk factor.

To reduce your risk of heart conditions or cardiovascular disease, it is important to monitor your overall health. Measure your cholesterol levels regularly as well as your blood pressure rate. Cholesterol tests will distinguish between your levels of bad cholesterol, good cholesterol, and triglycerides in the blood. High levels of bad cholesterol don't present with any physical symptoms, so the only way to manage it is by consistently checking your levels. Hypertension is also a major contributing risk factor for heart disease, and you will often experience very few symptoms before it is a major problem.

Hypertension

Hypertension or high blood pressure is common in women over 50. Hypertension can be passed down through the generations, but regular exercise, good nutrition, and weight-control can help you to avoid the development of high blood pressure. Blood pressure refers to the pressure that your blood exerts on the walls of your veins and arteries. This pressure must be kept at a stable level. Our blood pressure naturally fluctuates slightly during the day, but when that pressure remains too high for an extended period, damage can be caused in the blood vessels, which can cause cardiovascular disease, kidney disease, and strokes.

The DASH diet (Dietary Approaches to Stop Hypertension) has been designed specifically for those who suffer from high blood pressure. The DASH diet can be combined with fasting to multiply your chances of reducing your blood pressure and preventing hypertension. Your blood pressure reading consists of two numbers, a diastolic reading and a systolic reading. The systolic reading measures the pressure that your blood puts on your arteries when your heart beats and the diastolic reading reads the pressure inside the arteries between heart beats. The DASH diet is essentially a list of the foods which should be eaten and the frequency at which they should be eaten. In the DASH diet, it is recommended that sodium intake is limited to between 1,500 milligrams and 2,300 milligrams per day depending whether you are required to restrict sodium. At least two portions of low-fat dairy products and unsaturated fats are recommended as well as four portions each of fruit, vegetables, nuts, seeds, and legumes. The DASH diet also calls for at least six portions each of whole grains and lean animal protein.

In general, in order to follow these guidelines, you should include more vegetables, fruits, whole grains, and low-fat protein sources. The guidelines for this diet also recommend limiting alcohol units to one per week for women, and two units of alcohol per week, for men. The diet also recommends that sweets are limited to five portions per week (Ellis & Nall, 2017).

Cancer

Cancer is the growth of uncontrolled, abnormal cells. Instead of old cells dying they replicate and form new and abnormal cells. These abnormal cells group together into tumors or masses. Different types of cancer originate in various organs and areas of the body. These points of origination can include cervix, breasts, brain, liver, stomach, skin, and bones. Genetically predisposition has long been thought to be the biggest contributor to developing cancer yourself, but, in reality, only about five percent of cancer cases can be attributed to genetic causes. In the remaining cases, the causes of cancer are environmental and lifestyle factors. Physical inactivity, smoking cigarettes, poor nutrition, infections, air pollution, stress, alcohol, sun exposure, and excess weight are all far higher contributors to the development of cancer than genetics. Inflammation in the body is a precursor to cancer.

A lot of emphasis has been placed on searching our genomes for the clues to preventing chronic diseases. Craig Venter, a genome research expert, explains that this is misleading us because genes play such a small role. It is the environmental factors and the lifestyle factors that put us at risk for these diseases and we need to focus our energies on changing those.

A link between regional diet and cancer has been established. When we look at the common types and rates of cancers seen in various regions and compare that to how individuals who immigrated to different regions had their expectation of cancer impacted, there is a definite correlation. Asian countries have a rate of prostate cancer that is 25 percent lower than the global average and a rate of breast cancer that is at a 10 percent lower rate. When people of Asian origin moved to Western countries and made it their home for a significant period, eating the local diet, their rate of cancer incidence became the same as the Western country they had moved to.

Chronic alcohol abuse as well as sustained daily alcohol intake is also a risk factor for the development of cancer. The development of cancers of the esophagus, liver, larynx, oropharynx, and breasts are often linked with alcohol. Even occasional alcohol use when coexisting with other risk factors can still play a role in the development of cancer.

One of the most prominent contributing risk factors in the development of cancer, though, is diet, with approximately 35 percent of all cancer deaths showing a direct link to the patient's diet. Some cancers are impacted more by diet than other types. In cancers of the colon or rectal areas of the body about 70 percent of cases could directly be linked back to dietary factors. While we cannot yet determine exactly how food causes cancer or which are the main cancer-causing foods, we do know that most carcinogens are found in food additives, or the cooking process. Keep this in mind when we discuss the benefits of a raw diet later in this book (Anand, 2015).

There are several food groups that should be focused on in order to reduce the risk of cancer in women over 50. Cruciferous vegetables (a group of vegetables, which include broccoli, cauliflower, and kale) contain a plant compound called sulforaphane, which is believed to have powerful properties to prevent the development of cancer. Carrots can reduce the risk of lung, stomach, and prostate cancer, by up to 18 percent. Carrots are refreshing as a raw snack dipped in a fresh tzatziki dip or hummus or cooked as a delicious side dish with dinner. They are also great when juiced, raw, or with other vegetables and fruits. The high fiber levels in beans have been shown to decrease the risk of colonic and rectal cancers. Bilberries, raspberries, and blueberries slow down the spread of cancer and reduce the mass of the tumors.

Cinnamon has long been used in homeopathic medicine for its blood sugar stabilization properties as well as for the reduction in inflammation. This inflammation reduction is believed to also reduce the risk of cancer. A daily addition to your diet of one teaspoon of cinnamon may reduce your risk of developing throat and brain cancers. It is also shown to impact the spread and growth of tumors in people who already have a cancer diagnosis. Selenium-rich, Brazil nuts reduce the risk of lung cancer. Walnuts are also known to decrease the growth rate of tumors. Olive oil, when included as a regular part of the diet, brings a significant reduction in the risk of digestive system and breast cancers. Increase your intake of olive oil by using it in place of any other cooking or salad oils that you would ordinarily use.

Curcumin, well known for its anti-inflammatory effects, is the active ingredient in turmeric. It is also an antioxidant and has a positive impact on the risk of cancer. By adding three teaspoons of turmeric to your food per day, you can help reduce your risk of prostate, colon, brain, and throat cancers. In order to be absorbed in the body, it must be consumed with black pepper and an unsaturated fat (such as olive oil). The daily intake of Golden Paste is recommended by homeopaths. You can make Golden Paste at home by combining the following:

- one cup of water
- one-third of a cup of unsaturated fat (such as olive oil)

- three tablespoons of freshly cracked black pepper
- half a cup of turmeric

In a pan, mix the turmeric and water and stir until it reaches a boil. Remove from the stovetop and the oil and add the black pepper. After it has cooled, decant into a glass container with a tight seal lid. Store your Golden Paste in the fridge for up to three weeks, and take at least a quarter teaspoon per day.

The risk of colon, digestive system, and upper respiratory tract cancers is noticeably reduced when citrus fruits are eaten regularly. Flaxseed is high in fiber, so it is highly useful in reducing the incidence of digestive tract cancers. Include flaxseed in your diet daily by adding a tablespoon of it to smoothies, baked goods, or cereal.

Breast cancer is a highly complex cancer, and its origins and impetus are many and varied. Some foods have been shown to slow the progression of breast cancer and prevent its occurrence. These include soybeans and soybean-based products; fruits and vegetables; high fiber foods; turmeric and other foods with anti-inflammatory properties; low-fat dairy products; plant foods that contain high antioxidant levels; and foods that have high levels of vitamin D. A largely plant-based diet has been shown to reduce a woman's risk of developing breast cancer by 15 percent. Carrots, which are high in beta carotene, interferes with the growth of breast cancer cells. Excess estrogen can be a factor in the development of breast cancer, and fiber has been shown to help reduce the levels of estrogen in the body (Dresden, 2019).

Diabetes

Type 2 diabetes is very prevalent in women over 50 due to the belly fat deposits that are common after menopause. It is, therefore, important for us to understand the two types of diabetes, what causes each and how we can avoid them through the nutrition that we pair with fasting.

There are two forms of diabetes. The first, type 1 diabetes, is an auto-immune disease that occurs when your immune system confuses the beta cells of your pancreas, responsible for producing insulin, with diseased cells. This makes your immune system start destroying the beta cells, resulting in your body failing to produce its own insulin. Type 2 diabetes is the most common and is also related to your body's glucose levels, but it is not an auto-immune response. In type 2 diabetes, your body produces some insulin, but it does not use it in the way that it is supposed to. Although type 1 diabetes as an autoimmune disease can also be helped by fasting and nutrition, we will focus here on type 2 diabetes as this is the most common form identified in women over 50. Lifestyle factors such as diet, obesity, and physical inactivity are the predominant cause of type 2 diabetes and genetic risk factors also play a role. Type 2 diabetes starts with insulin resistance wherein the body starts incorrectly using insulin and produces more to compensate. Eventually, the pancreas starts to become overwhelmed and glucose levels will rise in the body, which marks the full development of type 2 diabetes (NIH, n.d.). Diabetics or those with pre-diabetes symptoms or risk factors should steer clear of any foods that are high in trans or saturated fats and fried foods. Stay away from any foods with high sodium or sugar levels. Beverages with high sugar content should be limited and only one unit of alcohol should be consumed per day. Portion sizing is a vital consideration for those with pre-diabetic symptoms and diagnosed diabetics. The plate portioning method works well. On a nine-inch dinner plate, split the plate into three portions. Half of the plate is for non-starchy vegetables. Within the remaining half, one half is for protein, and the other half is for starch, grain, or a starchy vegetable. You may need to count the carbohydrates you take in, depending on the severity of your diabetes (NIH, n.d.).

Brain Disease

While diseases like Alzheimer's and dementia are generally known to develop later in life, there is always the risk of early-onset development and it is important for women over 50 to understand the root causes of the various brain diseases and the way that nutrition can be paired with fasting to prevent and reduce the risk factors of developing these conditions.

Brain disease is a term that describes any disturbance of the activity in the brain or abnormal brain function that could result from disease or physical damage such as blunt force trauma. Dementia describes the loss of cognitive function, memory, and problem-solving skills. It usually occurs in old age. Alzheimer's is a disease of the brain and is often the cause of dementia.

Alzheimer's disease develops when the neural cells and pathways begin to stop functioning. While there is no cure for Alzheimer's disease, there is research being done suggesting that certain dietary exclusions and inclusions can slow the onset or even prevent it altogether depending on the other coexisting risk factors. Genetics can increase the risk of developing brain disease and alcohol use and smoking have also been shown to increase the risk. A build-up of plaque inside the lining of arteries called atherosclerosis, has an impact on the prevalence of dementia, as do chronically elevated bad cholesterol levels. Atherosclerosis can be limited by autophagy. Diabetes sufferers are known to have a higher risk of developing dementia (Stanford Health Care, n.d.). Nutrition evidently plays a major role in the development of brain disease. So much so that a specific diet has been developed to reduce the risk. The MIND diet recommends:

- Six servings (or more) of green, leafy vegetables including kale, spinach, and collards per week
- A salad every day as well as at least one other vegetable

- Five servings of nuts per week as the healthy fats, antioxidants, and fiber found in nuts is of great benefit to brain health.
- Blueberries and strawberries at least twice per week
- Beans, due to their high fat and protein content and low calorie count, should be eaten at least twice per week
- At least three servings per day of whole grains

The food groups to avoid include red meat, butter and margarine, cheese, pastries and sweets, and fried and fast foods (Cohen, 2015).

Maximize Your Health and Happiness After 50

Bone health is super important after the age of 50, as we know that estrogen plays a role in the processing of minerals like calcium and phosphorus, which are vital for bone health. While supplements are a good idea, there is no replacement for a well-rounded bone health diet. Soy is a surprising component of a healthy bone-strength diet. Soy products such as soy milk and tofu are highly beneficial and they help to limit your intake of animal products which, in excess, can lead to risk factors for cardiovascular disease. Excessive consumption of animal protein has also been thought to contribute to the development of Alzheimer's Disease. Although fasting does not impact muscle mass, the natural aging process does so you would be well-advised to up the amount of protein you take in. Again, plant-based proteins are always going to have far better health benefits than animal proteins over all, but you do need to eat more of a plant-based source to get in the same amount of protein so ensure that you are focusing on healthy proteins like lentils and tofu. When addressing your exercise regime to compensate for this natural muscle mass loss, you will also want to include more weight training exercises than you have before.

The importance of good quality sleep cannot be over-emphasized, and there is a surprising link between sleep disturbances like snoring and your heart health as a woman over 50. Snoring may be an indicator of a condition called obstructive sleep apnea which disrupts breathing during sleep. This erratic oxygen supply to the brain and other organs can contribute to heart disease much faster in women than it does in men. If you are struggling with snoring it is vital to understand the root cause and if it is sleep apnea, consider getting this treated with medication or surgery. Not only will you improve your quality of sleep (as well as your partner's!), you will help to reduce your risk of heart disease. While we are on the topic of sleep, it is also important to address your sleeping position. Studies have shown that sleeping on your side or stomach is more likely to cause wrinkles than if you sleep on your back. Of course, for those who snore, sleeping on your back makes it worse, so that's another reason to sort out your snoring so that you can change up your sleeping position. Despite what some will tell you, your sleep hours requirement does not decrease that significantly. After the age of 50 you still need at least seven to eight hours of sleep a night. An idea that may be beneficial in helping you to get the best sleep possible is setting a bedtime. Although this may sound a little like you are regressing to childhood, setting a bedtime helps you to structure your day (which is highly beneficial when fasting) and it gives you time to start unwinding and switching off electronic devices at least an hour before your bedtime.

Reducing sodium in your diet is a given but it is actually even more important for women than for men. Firstly, it reduces blood pressure and prevents hypertension far more effectively in women. This is, of course, also beneficial for kidney health as it puts less pressure on these organs to rid the body of waste salt.

Changes in the urinary tract after menopause can cause an increase in the urge to urinate as well as impact the efficacy of the bladder muscles to hold in urine until you are ready to release it. This form of incontinence as well as the urinary tract infections that often come with it, can be treated and there are medications, devices, and exercises that can help to limit the impact of this change on your life.

The link between our emotions and the way we experience menopause is proven, and studies have shown that women who live in abusive relationships or suffer from emotional disorders are highly likely to have a more severe experience of menopausal symptoms. This is the time to be enjoying your life and moving into a new phase with strength and independence. If you have lived in an abusive relationship for many years, perhaps now is the time to get out and give yourself the best opportunity to live a happy and healthy life after 50. It is also helpful to ensure that you keep up your relationships with friends during this time. You will need people to talk to who understand what you are going through and solid relationships are a boon for emotional stability.

The three most impactful risk factors for heart disease, besides obesity, are smoking, diabetes and high blood pressure. Female smokers are three times more likely to suffer from a heart attack than non-smokers.

While fasting will help to improve your immune responses, you may want to consider getting an annual flu vaccination if you are not already doing so. As we age and especially when our hormones are in flux, we do become more susceptible to disease. Our bodies are also not as primed to fight back as they ordinarily would be so the impact of a bout of flu that you could ordinarily beat down quite easily may hit you harder after the age of 50. Diet can play a role in improving your immune responses as well by including as much fresh produce as possible.

Our sight is another thing that changes quite drastically after the age of 50 and if you don't address it quickly you could end up with related problems like headaches, eye strain, and even car accidents if your vision deteriorates that much. It happens to everyone so there is no reason to be embarrassed or to try and pretend that it's not happening. Make an appointment with your optometrist and get yourself fitted with reading glasses or contact lenses. It will make your life far easier.

A concerted effort should be made to reduce your alcohol intake after the age of 50. In general women should limit their drinking to one alcoholic drink per day. Excessive alcohol consumption is not just bad for the liver but, in women, it is known to contribute to declined brain health, increased risk of breast cancer, as well as cardiovascular disease.

As we age, our body's capability to take the nutrients it needs from food changes and this can impact a wide range of areas health-wise. Vitamin B12 is quite severely impacted and this is made worse if you are on chronic medication. Vitamin B12 supplements are useful and monthly injections can also be helpful to increase energy levels and help level out your mood. Fiber intake should also be increased as you will also be absorbing less of this from your food than usual. Additional fiber will help to keep menopausal constipation at bay as well as the constipation that can result in your first few days of fasting. In general, your vitamin and mineral needs change after the age of 50. When your menstruation stops, for instance, you will need less folate and iron so your usual supplements may be doing more harm than good. Have a chat with your doctor about your specific vitamin and mineral needs after the age of 50 (Mann, 2019).

Plant-based medicines can be really beneficial in helping to stave off the unpleasant side effects of menopause. Essential oils are particularly useful and you should certainly consider investigating the benefits of alternative medicines. These products work well with fasting as both work with your body's natural processes. Add meditation and mindfulness to this and you will be packing a tool set of phenomenal power in your fight against the symptoms of menopause.

Chapter 6:
IF Methods and Modifications—Enjoy Them Safely

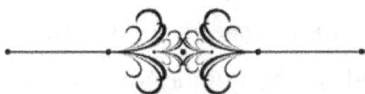

One of the best things about intermittent fasting is its flexibility. Unlike other regimes that may require you to eat very specific foods and follow strict guidelines, as long as you understand the principles of fasting, you can pretty much decide for yourself what works best for your personal situation.

In this chapter, we will cover all of the types of intermittent fasting methods that are available. We will also discuss which are best for perimenopausal, menopausal and post-menopausal women. With this information in hand, you can then decide for yourself, which method will best suit you. You may need to try a few different methods first in order to determine the best fit for your lifestyle.

Intermittent fasting methods are differentiated primarily by the period of time (in hours) allocated to fasting and eating respectively. Certain methods are differentiated by the number of days in the week on which you fast. These fasting methods have also been adapted and slightly converted, in the past, by diet professionals into branded regimes. We will also clarify these adapted fasting regimes to ensure that you understand how the simply fasting method has been changed to fit the branded method.

While intermittent fasting does not require that you restrict calories, if you are wanting to lose weight, certain methods do make suggestions for restriction of calories in the eating window. It must be noted that you do not need to restrict calories in order to receive the benefits of intermittent fasting. If you already eat a healthy diet, you may only need to increase your activity level and combine it with fasting in order to lose a small amount of weight.

Sarah L. Moore

5:2 Twice-a-Week Fasting

In this method, the numbers mentioned denote the numbers of days in the week on which you fast and not the number of hours in a day, as is usually the case. This method involves calorie restriction and suggests that on two days of the week, you should restrict your calories to 500 calories (a 200 calorie meal and a 300 calorie meal) during your eating window. This means that you will combine this method with an hour-based fasting method such as 16:8, for instance. It is not advisable to do this on consecutive days, so if you decide to fast on a Monday, then fast again on a Wednesday or Thursday. On your non-fasting days, your diet should be as close to normal as possible keeping in mind that fasting is not a ticket to binge on junk food. Always maintain a healthy and balanced diet that includes plenty of fruit and vegetables.

Alternate Day Fasting

This method, again, focuses on the days in the week that you will fast. It does not limit you to only two days in the week but does require that you have a break day between fasts. This is very important for women who have not yet entered menopause or women who are perimenopausal and still experiencing menstruation. If you are calorie restricting—and it is key to note that this is only required if you wish to lose weight—it is recommended that on your fast days you only consume around 500 calories in your eating window. On your break days, you should eat your normal, healthy diet. Again, this method would be combined with one of the hourly methods such as 16:8.

16:8 Fast

This method denotes the number of hours in a day that you should allocate to a fasting window and an eating window respectively. The first number is the number of hours in the fast (16) and the second number is the number of hours in the eating window (8). During the fast you will only drink beverages that do not have a calorie content. The easiest way to implement this fasting method is as a continuation of the natural fast you undertake while sleeping. If you are getting your required hours of sleep then you are already fasting for eight hours, you can then wake up and simply continue that for another eight hours. This is really the most convenient way of fasting as the only meal you are missing is breakfast. This method is also the safest for women and you can work your way up to 16 hours if it is a bit difficult to do in one chunk to begin with. This method should then be combined with one of the weekly allocations. Your best bet is alternate day fasting although starting on a 5:2 method might be preferable to begin with and then you can work your way up to more days in the week if you prefer. Always give yourself a break day in between.

14:10 and 12:12 Fasts

These methods are also denoted by hours in the day and are really just a variation on the 16:8 method. Starting on the 12-hour fast might be easier for beginners and, really, you can start at any time increment and work your way up. The key is to make sure that you succeed so if, for you, slow and steady wins the race, then that is what you should do. Keep in mind that ketosis (fat burning) starts anywhere between 12 and 16 hours after your last meal and this depends on your fitness level, activity level and how many stores of glucose you have to burn off before your body gets to the fat. If you are obese and inactive, you will not see fat burning results at a 10 hour fast so your calorie intake will need to be more restricted and your activity levels will need to increase significantly.

The 24-Hour Fast

From the outset it is important to note that this method is not recommended for women due to the impact it may have on our hormonal balance. Some women are able to successfully use this method but it should only be tried with careful consideration. The method involves fasting for a full 24-hours, once or twice a week. Most people that use this method will fast from meal to meal, for instance breakfast to breakfast.

The side effects experienced with intermittent fasting are particularly severe on a 24-hour fast so if you are going to try it, rather do so after you have already made your body accustomed to fasting with the 16:8 method or similar. On the days that you are not fasting, you should eat your normal, healthy diet (Health Essentials, n.d.).

The Warrior Diet

This method of fasting is an adaptation by fitness and nutrition expert, Ori Hofmekler. It is based on the eating patterns of ancient soldiers who would consume nothing during the day while in battle and then feast at night. Hofmekler acknowledges that this method is based on his beliefs and not necessarily on scientific information. The fast component of the method, of course, does have scientific backing but, its extended duration is not suitable for most women. The Warrior method suggests fasting completely or undereating for 20 hours of the day and then eating as much food as you want at night. Hofmekler's specific plan does not insist upon true fasting and does allow for raw fruits and vegetables as well as boiled eggs to be eaten during the fast window, if required.

While many swear by this method, it should certainly be approached with caution as the almost binge-like method of breaking a significantly long fast can lead to serious digestive and sleep problems (Kubala, 2018).

Choosing a Method

No one can tell you which is the right method of intermittent fasting for you. The choice is based on your individual situation, your body type, health status, and many other considerations. With the knowledge that you are gaining, you will likely have a good idea of which methods will be suitable for you to try. The easiest and safest way of determining this is by starting small and working your way up. Most of us are already starting off a base fast of eight hours while we are sleeping. So the best way to work your way up is to slowly increase your fast hours from that base every few days. On the first few occasions you fast, you can start at nine hours, then 10 and so on until you feel that you have reached your "sweet spot." Determining this point is finding the line between feeling well while still burning fat and activating the other benefits of fasting and pushing yourself sufficiently to ensure you are getting as much as you can out of fasting. Although fasting will not permanently damage your body even if you did decide to do 24-hour fasts, your health should always be your first priority. That is, after all, why you started this journey in the first place. If you are fasting with a friend or as part of a support group, do not make the mistake of comparing your fasting journey to anyone else's. As each person is unique, there is no way to compare the progress of one person to another. If you are a competitive type, make the competition with yourself and push yourself a little more every day.

Tips for Maintaining Fasting

Fasting is not difficult but it does take focus and the willingness to put some hard work in to get yourself to the goal. As we have mentioned, there are some side effects that you may experience right at the start of your fasting journey. None of these should be so severe that you can't deal with them by planning ahead. This is also why we recommend that you start small and work your way up so that you don't experience all of the side effects at once or at an intense level.

There are a few ways that you can improve your chances of maintaining your fast. One of the most important factors is to ensure that you remain well-hydrated. We can often mistake thirst for hunger, so when you believe that you are feeling hungry, try a glass of water instead. The action of drinking the water helps to keep your mind off the hunger, it fills you up temporarily and by staying hydrated you can avoid headaches, which often occur in the beginning of your fasting journey. If you experience significant brain fog initially, you should also check your hydration levels as this can be as a result of being dehydrated.

Do your best not to obsess about the fact that you are not eating. Our minds play tricks on us and even though we may usually miss breakfast quite naturally, when we are regimenting this skipped meal, our brain suddenly turns it into a major problem. Keep in mind that your hunger will be sated extremely easily. In fact, just one mouthful of food will already start reducing those pangs of hunger but that same mouthful of food stops you from enjoying the benefits of fasting that are starting to occur in your body at that time. Again, this is another good reason to build up to your ideal fast duration rather than going right into it from day one. Remind yourself when you wake up that you have already fasted for eight hours, then ask yourself if you can do just one more hour? Then, can you do just one more? If you continue on in this vein, you will be able to build on your successes and easily master fasting. If you think that you are going to struggle with your first few initial fasts, plan something to do that will distract you.

Eat foods during your eating window that will fill you up and give you sustained energy as this will make your fasting period far easier (Leonard, 2020).

Planning ahead for your eating window can be an extremely powerful way to ensure that you maintain your fast. Food preparation, in advance, can help you to avoid the panic of trying to find something to break your fast with. It is this meal that is absolutely imperative to plan for as, if you don't, you can end up ruining a lot of your hard work by binging or eating whatever junk food is at hand. Whether you work from home or outside of the home, have a plan for what you are going to eat to break your fast. Prepare sandwich fillings ahead of time or freeze soups and broths so that you always have something ready. You can have all of your smoothie ingredients chopped up and ready to go in a container. Then, when you are ready to end your fasting window simply pop it in the food processor and enjoy. Batch cooking is a good way to prepare in advance for meals. When you cook at night, try to cook twice the amount that you are going to eat in that sitting and freeze the rest for other meals. If you roast a chicken, use that time and electricity to roast a second chicken at the same time, then you can shred it and freeze the meat for sandwiches wraps and salads.

Be mindful during your journey. Listen to what your body and your mind is saying and work with that. Fasting is a great way to really get to know yourself and you may be surprised by the actual relationship you have with food.

If you struggle with headaches or feeling light headed, try putting a small pinch of salt on your tongue or in your water. This helps to give you the electrolytes that you might be missing. Don't overdo it on the salt though.

If you are struggling with constipation in the first few days, hydration, yogurts and high fiber foods are your friends. This should sort itself out after a few days but if you are still struggling, you can also take a mild laxative.

In summary, The following tips may help people stay on track and maximize the benefits of intermittent fasting. Keep hydrated. Drink a lot of water and drinks with no calories, such as herbal teas, throughout the day. Green tea is a great beverage option for fasting. Catechins and polyphenols are natural compounds found in all tea plants but are in high concentrations in green tea. Catechins reduce cell damage by being natural antioxidants. Polyphenols are micronutrients that aid in the prevention of heart disease as well as neurodegenerative disease, digestive issues, and diabetes. If green tea is not to your taste, you can try a product made with the entire green tea leaf, called matcha, as it has a slightly different flavor.

Don't obsess over food. Plan distractions on fasting days to stop thinking about food. Rest and relax. Avoid exhausting activities on fasting days, but light exercise like Pilates or yoga may be beneficial. Make each calorie count. If the chosen plan allows some calories during fasting periods, select foods that are nutrient-dense and rich in protein, fiber, and healthy fats, like beans, lentils, eggs, fish, nuts, and avocado. Eat high-volume foods. Select filling but low-calorie foods, like popcorn, raw vegetables, and fruits with high water content, such as grapes and melon. Increase the taste without the calories. Season meals liberally with garlic, herbs, spices, or vinegar. These are very low in calories but full of flavor, to help reduce feelings of deprivation. Choose nutrient-dense foods after the fasting period. Eating foods that are high in fiber, vitamins, minerals, and other nutrients helps to keep blood sugar levels steady and prevent nutrient deficiencies. A balanced diet will also contribute to weight loss and overall health.

We are thrilled to hear you and your friends are **enjoying my writing! Please** let us know **by reviewing the book on Amazon.com,**

If you have any questions to clarify or something that you are enjoying, do not hesitate to write on the review, it will help me for the next book.

Or you can even visit us at athenapublications.com and be updated on my new arrivals and special promotions,

Chapter 7:
Don't Do That! Do This Instead

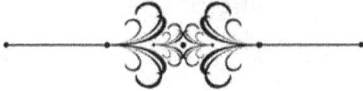

A lthough intermittent fasting is really flexible and possibly one of the easiest lifestyle regimes to undertake, it is also easy to make mistakes that could end up costing you some of the benefits you should be receiving. Most of these mistakes will revolve around the way we behave in our eating window. While fasting does not dictate which foods you should eat, there are certainly foods which make it easier for us to maintain a fast.

Common Fasting Mistakes

Fasting is not a free pass to binge on as many unhealthy snacks as you want during your eating window. Trying to use intermittent fasting to improve your health while still eating processed, junk food in huge quantities is like trying to put out a fire with a bucket of water while alternately spiking it with gas from the other end. It's pointless. It is not necessary for you to completely avoid all of your favorite foods forever, and a burger now and then is not going to harm anyone but it cannot be a continuous part of your diet and you also should definitely not be binging. Take-out meals are designed for binging. You know very well that just a burger would fill you up but food companies design meals to be supersized and to add fries and fizzy, sugar-laden drinks. They then incentivize this larger purchase by making it cheaper to purchase a whole meal than just a single burger. If you base your food choices on the marketing that is spewed out by food corporations then you are setting yourself up for trouble and no amount of fasting will fix the damage you will do to your body.

The process of autophagy means that your body is breaking down damaged portions and using that to rebuild healthier structures. That also means that your body becomes more sensitive to the type of food you put into it. Foods that are dense in calories will only cause your body to crave more calories. Instead, focus on a diet that is predominantly made up of whole foods and plenty of fruit and vegetables, and if you absolutely must have a processed or take-out meal, don't fall for the supersize option.

In certain sections of this book we have discussed the concept of calorie restricting during the eating window if you are fasting to lose weight. Interestingly, this is not always necessary, especially if you only have a small amount of weight to lose. It can also lead to another common mistake in fasting and that is restricting your calories too severely. Keep in mind that you are now restricting your eating to a very specific window, where before, you likely snacked for a lot of the day and you may not have realized how many calories you were actually taking in. If you are wanting to lose weight through fasting try to track your normal eating for a few days before you begin fasting and keep a record of how many calories you consumed. Then, when you start fasting compare that to how many calories you are now taking in during your eating window without imposing any restrictions. You will likely already notice a significant difference and by combining this with exercise, there may be no further need for restriction. The problem with significantly reducing your calorie consumption is that you also decrease your nutrient consumption and this can lead to problems further down the line.

We have already recommended a slow and steady start to your fasting journey and it should be noted that trying to do too much too soon is also another reason that many people fail at fasting. If you are generally not living a healthy lifestyle and you are not physically fit, attempting to start a rigorous training regime, restrict calories, and fast at the same time is going to be catastrophic, and really it is just putting unnecessary stress on your body. Rather than trying to do everything at once, start small with a few things and then add as you go, you'll find the process a lot easier and you will be far more successful in the long term. When deciding which fasting method you are going to go with and the rate at which you are going to move yourself towards that window, you need to get a good idea of how often you eat now. As with measuring your calories, you may really have no idea how often you eat either as in your memory, 'eating' means sitting down for a meal but you may very well be eating as often as every three hours. Once you have determined how often you eat now, you can start stretching yourself out slowly.

While, in the beginning, you will want to ensure that you stick to your fasting and eating windows, the true joy of fasting is that it is reteaching your body to understand when it really needs food. If you are able to continue with your fasting journey for long enough, you will understand the shift. Your body will no longer give you false signals of hunger and you will be able to tell the difference between real hunger and mind tricks. When this happens, you won't have to worry about the clock anymore because your body will be set into a natural eating cycle.

Drinking water is not just important for hydration, it also helps your body to move out the toxins that are being produced as by-products of the cleansing process it is undergoing. Keep hydrated constantly and use water as your new 'snack' (Lowery, 2019).

Binging at the end of a fast is a very common mistake. In the beginning, until your body figures out what it's supposed to be doing, you are very likely to be pretty hungry by the time your fasting window ends and it is very tempting to 'justify' your binge with the fact that you have just fasted for 16 hours. If you are trying to lose weight, you are shooting yourself in the foot, and even if you are not trying to lose weight, you are going to end up feeling ill. Instead, break your fast with a light and nutritious meal and plan ahead so that, no matter where you are, you have such a meal at hand to break your fast with. People who are fasting for extended periods of time (72 hours or more) need to be very careful about how they reintroduce food. Although we do not recommend extended fasting for women, it is important to understand how dangerous binge eating can be after an extended fast. Refeeding syndrome is a set of physical complications that results from someone who has not eaten for a long period of time, suddenly gorging on food. Refeeding syndrome can result in hospitalization and even death if not carefully monitored. This is why you will find that people who have not been able to eat solid food for a long period of time are slowly reintroduced to solid food and not immediately given a huge plate of food.

The opposite of binging is when you don't eat enough during your eating window. If you don't have a large amount of weight to lose, there is no need to restrict your calories. If you go too far down the calorie restriction route, you will end up making yourself ill. By the same token, you need to ensure that you focus on what you are eating to ensure that you are taking in the required nutrients.

A common mistake during the fasting window is drinking beverages with hidden calories in them which essentially end up breaking your fast and slowing the autophagy process. If you are drinking coffee or tea, it has to be black and sugarless. Even a splash of milk or sweetener will halt your fast because they contain calories. Many people think that because diet soda doesn't have sugar in it that it is okay to drink while fasting and that is incorrect. Despite not having sugar, it still contains calories. Even products that claim to be 'zero-calorie,' still have an impact on insulin levels and therefore break your fast.

Fasting is going to be a whole lot easier if you don't have to plan your life around it and thankfully, its flexible nature means that you don't have to miss out on social events with friends or dinner with your partner because it clashes with your fast. You can simply move your fast to a more convenient time and pick it up where you left off. No harm done (Fields, 2019).

One of the easiest ways to make fasting difficult for yourself is by simply choosing the wrong method for your lifestyle. You know your own life better than anyone else. You know your family, your job, and your own personal habits. Do not pick a fasting method that is going to completely go against your day-to-day life. Instead, find one (or create one) that is right for you.

Fasting-Friendly Foods

Intermittent fasting eating can be confusing. This is because fasting is an eating pattern not a diet plan. Fasting does not dictate what foods can be included in your diet but tells you about when to eat. A lack of clear dietary guidelines can give an incorrect idea that

Sarah L. Moore

you can eat whatever you wish. For others, this makes it difficult to choose suitable foods and drinks. This can not only undermine your weight-loss efforts but can also make you more likely to be under or overnourished. Eating during fasting is focused on health and not just losing weight. Therefore, it is very important to choose foods that are dense in nutrients such as fruits, vegetables, lean proteins, and healthy fats.

While you can really eat anything you please during your eating window, there are definitely foods to avoid and foods to choose if you want to increase your chances of being successful in your fasting journey. Remember that when you fast and promote autophagy your body is clearing out all of the damaged parts and it needs proper nutrition in order to do that and to build healthy news cells. The ideal scenario is to take in nutrient-dense foods, such as whole-wheat bread, which when compared to white bread, is far higher in potassium, magnesium, and zinc. Leafy greens like spinach and kale and whole grains like barley and quinoa are extremely nutrient dense. Macronutrient levels must be monitored to ensure that you are giving your body what it needs in order to carry out its

123

normal processes but also to perform the tasks associated with fasting. The nutritional compounds that your body utilizes to perform different functions are called macronutrients. The three major macronutrients are protein, carbohydrates, and fats. Your body uses protein to support the organ functioning and the building of new tissue in organs that regenerate. Your body uses carbohydrates as an energy source in the form of glucose. Fat is important in maintaining the balance of your hormone levels, keeping skin and hair healthy, and insulating nerves. Fats also serve as a reserve energy source (Tendall, 2018).

The World Health Organization links good nutrition to, amongst others, lower risk of chronic diseases such as diabetes and cardiovascular disease, a stronger immune system, and increased longevity. We tend to associate the words "poor nutrition" to the idea of people starving in poorer countries, but the reality is that poor nutrition is actually just a suboptimal level of nutrition. This means it is both overconsumption of the wrong foods and malnutrition due to an inability to access the right foods. People can, therefore, be overweight or underweight when suffering from poor nutrition. Even a person without any visible weight concerns can still be suffering from below par nutrition. The symptoms of these poor eating habits are just evident in different areas of their body. A weight within the acceptable range could put you at higher risk of non-communicable disease as if your poor nutrition habits are not visible they may not be attended to until it is too late.

The food we eat eventually becomes a part of us, as it integrates into our cellular structures. If you eat food that is easily integrated, your body will have an easier time digesting and using the fuel. If we eat poor quality food that is not healthy for you on an ongoing basis, your bodies will find it more and more difficult to break it down and rid your body of the waste. This additional strain on your body can be a contributing factor to the eventual occurrence of chronic disease.

There are foods that have been shown to positively impact levels of triglycerides, cholesterol, blood pressure, and inflammation and it is really important for us as women over 50 to understand which foods are helpful for which conditions so that when we fast, we can structure our eating window to include the most nutritious foods.

Kale, collards, and spinach are green, leafy vegetables that are excellent sources of vitamins, minerals, and antioxidants. They can be eaten cooked as a side, used in a salad, or liquidized into a smoothie. The antioxidant action inhibits the process that releases cell-damaging free radicals into the body. Vitamin K is the vitamin that helps to reduce the risk factors for heart disease. It helps to clot blood and protect the arteries. These vegetables are also high in dietary nitrates and help to promote health of arteries and reduce hypertension.

When choosing your grains, you definitely want to choose whole grains over refined grains as the additional fiber present in whole grains helps to reduce levels of bad cholesterol and decrease the risk of cardiovascular disease overall. A whole grain has three sections: the germ, the endosperm, and the bran. All three of these sections are rich in nutrients. When the germ and the bran portions are removed in the refining process, the nutrient value is significantly reduced. This refining also impacts the positive role it plays in your digestive tract. Examples of whole grains include buckwheat, oats, rye, barley, brown rice, and quinoa.

Berries are rich in anthocyanins, which are powerful antioxidants contributing towards lower free radical damage in the body. When making your smoothies, be sure to include berries. Frozen berries are just as nutritious as fresh berries so you can keep a constant supply in the freezer.

When cooking, always try to include some garlic in your food. Its taste isn't even noticeable in small amounts. Used in homeopathic remedies for centuries, garlic has been recommended as a treatment for many health issues. A compound called allicin, which garlic contains, is a powerful part of a healthy heart diet. Garlic inhibits the build-up of platelets and stabilizes blood pressure, which helps to prevent the formation of embolisms, clots, and the occurrence of strokes. Raw garlic is most powerful but if you prefer it in cooked food, crush the peeled clove and let it stand for a minute or two to build up the allicin levels.

Recommended Protein Sources

While long-term health is far better supported by plant-based proteins than animal-derived proteins, it does take a lot more quantity-wise of plant-based proteins to make up the same amount of protein from an animal source. Your healthiest bet will always be plant-based proteins but, here, we will cover both.

One of the most common global nutritional deficiencies is protein deficiency, as many people do not get enough of this macronutrient in their daily diet. This problem is most common in countries with food insecurities due to depressed economies. On the contrary, people are often consuming too much protein (often animal protein), in developed countries such as the US. As saturated fats are often a part of the food package with the protein content, this has a further negative impact on health.

In general you will require 0.8 grams of protein per kilogram of body weight. This will differ slightly depending on your activity levels and the type of exercise that you are doing. As we age, we also need more protein in our diet to make up for natural muscle mass loss. Protein is an important part of a fasting eating regime as it helps you to feel fuller for longer and boosts your metabolism. The following are the recommended sources of protein for fasting:

- Whole grains
- Beans
- Legumes
- Seeds
- Nuts
- Soy
- Seafood
- Eggs
- Poultry
- Fish
- Dairy products (yogurt, cheese, and milk)

Recommended Carbohydrate Sources

Carbohydrates are the major source of energy for your body and it is recommended that up to 65 percent of your daily calories should come from carbohydrates. Included under the carbohydrate umbrella are starch, fiber, and sugar. There are many eating plans that recommend cutting out carbohydrates completely, and this has led to the belief that carbohydrates cause weight gain. This is, of course, not true but anything in excess will cause problems and as a modern society we have started leaning toward carbohydrates that are high in sugar and low in fiber, which is the root of the problem. Even the keto diet, which recommends low carbohydrate consumption does not suggest that they should be completely removed from a balanced diet. The key is to aim for carbohydrate sources that are high in fiber as this helps us to lose and maintain weight, improve our glucose levels and lower blood pressure. The following foods are recommended sources of good carbohydrates when you are fasting:

- Chickpeas
- Beetroots
- Mangoes
- Kidney beans
- Avocado
- Brussels sprouts
- Carrots
- Almonds
- Chia seeds
- Broccoli
- Berries

- Oats
- Brown rice
- Quinoa
- Bananas

Recommended Fat Sources

Fats have as bad of a reputation as carbohydrates do, and it is just as unwarranted. Not all fats are bad for you. Fats are divided into two types: saturated and unsaturated fats. The difference in composition between fats is in the fatty acid molecules and how many have at least one molecular bond between them. Unsaturated fats are good for you and can reduce the risk of cardiovascular disease, high blood pressure, and the level of triglycerides in the bloodstream. Examples of unsaturated fats include peanut oil, canola oil, sunflower oil, and olive oil. Saturated fats, which are bad for you, reduce the levels of good cholesterol in your blood and increase bad cholesterol. Saturated fats are found in fried foods. The following are examples of sources of good fats, which are recommended for fasting:

- Chia seeds

- Extra virgin olive oil
- Full-fat yogurt
- Avocados
- Nuts
- Whole eggs
- Cheese
- Dark chocolate

While fish (particularly salmon) has the highest amount of good fats, if you don't enjoy fish, or if you are vegan or vegetarian, you can still get omega-3 from other sources, such as hemp. Hemp seeds contain an amino acid called arginine, which decreases certain inflammation markers in the body.

Chocolate might be a surprising item to see on a list of foods with health benefits, but dark chocolate with at least 70 percent cocoa content is a very healthy choice in small portions. Dark chocolate actually has similar antioxidant benefits to fruits like berries, and slows the oxidation process.

We should shift our focus on fats to choose the type of fat rather than the quantity. When manufacturers remove fat from a product to manufacture products that are labeled 'low-fat,' they will often replace the fat with refined carbohydrates. Due to the fact that our bodies digest carbohydrates much quicker than fat, this leads to changes in blood sugar, feeling more hungry, more quickly and weight gain (The Nutrition Source, n.d.). Obesity rates have increased hugely during the low-fat diet push we've been seeing for many years in food marketing.

Recommended Foods for Gut Health During Fasting

Your gut has a surprising connection to your immune system and it stems from billions of bacteria that live in your gut—microbiota. They help to send signals to your immune system about the type of pathogens to look out for, they also aid in maintaining gut health, digestion and they even play a role in mental health. When we are intermittent fasting it is vital not to put our microbiota out of sync. The following foods should therefore be included when fasting:

- Miso
- Kefir
- All vegetables
- Kombucha

- Fermented vegetables
- Tempeh
- Sauerkraut

Our gut microbiota first have contact with our immune system when we are born. From that first contact, they begin a mutualistic interaction where the microbiota regulate responses of parts of the immune system and, in turn, the immune system impacts the composition of gut microbiota. The intestinal wall forms a barrier preventing gut microbiota from leaking out into our body. This barrier still allows for interaction with the immune system though. The nutrients we take in as part of our diet feed our gut microbiota, and then, in return, they help us to digest the food we eat. Our diet, therefore, plays a role in how well the gut microbiota are able to perform their function. High levels of extremely energy-dense foods, animal proteins, saturated fats, simple sugars, high amounts of sodium, and not enough plant material, are all linked to disorders of the immune system. Metabolic products that directly interact with our bodies are produced by microbes. There is constant monitoring by the immune system of the condition of the gut microbiota and it utilizes that information to instruct other organs in the body in amending their functions to compensate. This balance can be disturbed by antibiotics, diet, and stress. Serious imbalances in gut microbiota can lead to chronic inflammation and the development of autoimmune diseases (Adaes, 2019).

Foods Recommended to Maintain Hydration

We get a surprising amount of water from the food we eat so when we change our eating schedule, we put ourselves at risk for dehydration. This can be remedied by eating food with a high water content during our eating window and ensuring that we get enough fluids in while we are fasting. Women need approximately 2.7 liters of water per day, depending on activity level and the environmental conditions. The following are good sources of hydration:

- Strawberries
- Watermelon
- Cantaloupe
- Oranges
- Black tea or coffee

- Lettuce
- Plain yogurt
- Skim milk
- Celery
- Cucumber
- Plain and sparkling water
- Tomatoes

Foods to Avoid When Intermittent Fasting

- Processed foods and meats
- Refined grains
- Saturated fats
- Alcoholic beverages
- Candy
- Sugary drinks (Shahzad, 2020)

Foods That Support Hormonal Health

In addition to the support that fasting offers in supporting hormonal health, there are also certain foods, that when included in your diet can help to even out any negative side effects from hormonal imbalances. These foods are appropriate for any hormonal issues including puberty, PMS, and the various stages of menopause. The secretion of hormones is also impacted by the foods we eat, specifically by the macronutrients contained in them. Foods that are high in macronutrients support the correct secretion and level maintenance of hormones. Foods that are high in sugar and alcohol can have a negative impact on your hormones. The following foods are good for improving hormonal health:

- **Avocado:** this source of unsaturated fat is not only very filling and great for your heart health but they are also loaded with beta-sitosterol which has an effect on estrogen, progesterone, and cortisol.

- **Flaxseed:** this source of omega-3 fatty acids also contains a significant amount of fiber and antioxidants. Flaxseed contain lignans which have an effect on estrogen and may offer protection against certain cancers.

- **Broccoli:** this member of the cruciferous family of vegetables because it is such an excellent source of calcium it helps to allay the symptoms of premenstrual syndrome by impacting estrogen levels. Other cruciferous vegetables include cauliflower, bok choy, Brussels sprouts, turnips, kale, and cabbage.

- **Pomegranate:** packed with antioxidants, this fruit can help block the production of excess estrogen in the body. Certain cancers respond to estrogen so they are reduced in risk by the regular consumption of pomegranate.

- **Salmon:** the high omega-3 content of this fish aids in cell-to-cell communication around hormonal secretion. It also improves mood, cognition, and heart health. Other similar sources include mackerel, lake trout, sardines, albacore tuna, and herring.

- **Leafy greens:** spinach, collard greens, beet greens, swiss chard, dandelion greens, and kale are packed with antioxidants which reduce inflammation and help to regulate estrogen and cortisol levels. They are also all great sources of iron which, when deficient, can lead to brain fog, headaches, and fatigue.

- **Nuts:** including almonds and walnuts are known to have a positive impact on the endocrine system, which is responsible for the control of hormones. Other positive impacts from eating nuts include lowering of insulin, maintenance of blood sugar, and protection of the cardiovascular system.

- **Soy:** soy products like edamame and tofu can have estrogen-like effects on the body in menopausal women and have been shown to assist in the reduction of hot flashes. Soy is also known to reduce the risk of breast cancer.

- **Turmeric:** this flavorful, yellow spice contains curcumin which is known to mimic the activity of estrogen. It is also an excellent anti-inflammatory and according to a 2009 study, provides as much relief to those with arthritis as chemical pain relievers. Turmeric root can help to minimize menstrual cramps.

- **Quinoa:** this complex-carbohydrate helps maintain sugar levels and therefore, keeps insulin and androgen level steady (Wolff, 2019).

Isoflavones are a class of flavonoids found in soy products. They provide many health benefits, including fighting osteoporosis, strengthening the cardiovascular system, improving cognitive function, and reducing the risk of hormone-related cancers by mimicking the hormone estrogen. Edamames, which are an immature form of soybeans, are very high in isoflavones. The beans are a staple in Asian diets, but they have also exploded in popularity in the West and edamame is now grown in the US. Poke bowls are a new fad food that contain edamame as a staple accompanied by a range of other carefully selected high-nutrition foods.

Raw Food Diet

An interesting option for women over 50 is switching to a raw food diet. A raw food diet is predominantly made up of unprocessed, whole plant-based, and organic foods. About three quarters of the diet should be uncooked. While some raw food dieters are vegan, many also eat raw meat and other animal products. If you are interested in trying a raw food diet, the following are some of the items you can eat:

- dried fruits
- soaked beans, legumes, and grains
- fresh fruit and vegetable juices
- coconut milk
- nut milk

- raw nut butters
- raw nuts and seeds
- purified water
- sun-dried fruits
- seaweeds
- fermented foods

On a raw food diet, the only heating that is allowed is with a dehydrator which is essentially hot air that never exceeds 115 degrees Fahrenheit. Some examples of raw meals include:

Fruit with dehydrated seeds for breakfast; apple with nut salad and stuffed large mushrooms. Raw foodists even have a chocolate chip recipe which involves grinding cashews and oats in a blender to make the dough then mixing coconut oil, cocoa powder and carob to make the chocolate chips and then combining and freezing for 30 minutes.

A body fed on a raw food diet is thought to be in a better position to prevent and fight disease. Certain vitamins are reduced or destroyed by cooking, so when these foods are eaten raw, we take in a greater number of nutrients. The food enzymes in food are destroyed above 116 degrees Fahrenheit. Raw food is also easier to digest than cooked food.

Those following a raw food diet claim to experience clearer skin, more energy, better digestion, weight loss, and lower risk of cardiovascular disease. Studies have indicated that a plant-based diet can be beneficial in weight loss and also reduce the risk of cardiovascular disease, cancer, obesity, and type 2 diabetes.

There is no harm in trying a raw food diet but we do recommend that you stick to a plant-based diet if you do so. Also watch out for the following possibly harmful elements when raw:

- Cassava: certain type are toxic
- Kidney beans: contain a chemical called phytohaemagglutinin, when consumed raw can be toxic.
- Buckwheat: green buckwheat is toxic. When juiced or eaten in large amounts it can be harmful, specifically to people with fair skin as it triggers photosensitivity and other skin issues.
- Pea seeds: grass peas, Khesari dal or almorta pea variants may cause lathyrism which is

weakness of the lower limbs caused by a neurological weakness.

- Parsnips: contain a chemical produced by plants as a defense mechanism against predators. This chemical is called furanocoumarin and is toxic to humans.

- Apricot kernels: contain amygdalin, which contains cyanide.

Certain vegetables are actually more beneficial when cooked. Tomatoes for instance increase in levels of the antioxidant lycopene when cooked, but cooking destroys its levels of vitamin C.

Anecdotal evidence suggests that people eating a raw food diet may well experience sustained weight loss, clearer skin, more energy, and a reduction in cholesterol and triglycerides in blood tests.

There are some considerations to make when deciding whether you will try a raw food diet in addition to intermittent fasting:

- It can be difficult to stick to this diet when you are outside of the home.

- Initial digestive problems may arise as your body gets used to raw food.

- If you don't actually need to lose weight, you will need to work hard to maintain your calorie count.

- A significant amount of discipline, organization, and preparation is required to keep up with this diet.

- You may be at risk of not getting sufficient vitamin B12, iron, calcium, fatty acids, protein, and vitamin D.

- Some raw food dieters have shown lower bone mass, although other than that their bones appeared healthy.

The best halfway point between a full raw diet and a standard cooked diet is to highly increase the intake of fresh, raw fruit, and vegetables (Brazier, 2017).

Combining Fasting and Keto or Vegetarian Diet

Some believe that combining fasting with certain eating plans such as a vegetarian or keto diet is more efficient for weight loss. There is evidence for and against this.

If you want to try a blend of fasting and the keto diet? Ensure that you are eating the following foods for a low-carb, high-fat diet, intermittent fasting food list:

Seventy-five percent of your daily calories from fats:

- Dark chocolate
- Fatty fish
- Avocados
- Chia seeds
- Extra virgin olive oil
- Nuts
- Cheese
- Whole eggs
- Full-fat yogurt

Twenty percent of your daily calories from protein:

- Soy
- Dairy products such as milk, yogurt, and cheese
- Poultry and fish
- Seeds and nuts

- Beans and legumes
- Seafood
- Eggs
- Whole grains

Five percent of your daily calories come from carbohydrates:

- Quinoa
- Oats
- Sweet potatoes
- Beetroots
- Brown rice

If you want to try blending a vegetarian diet with fasting, you can include the following:

For protein:

- Beans and legumes
- Soy
- Dairy products such as milk, yogurt, and cheese
- Whole grains
- Seeds and nuts

For carbohydrates:

- Sweet potatoes
- Avocado
- Carrots
- Broccoli
- Brussels sprouts
- Beetroot
- Chickpeas
- Quinoa
- Chia seeds
- Oats
- Brown rice
- Almonds
- Bananas
- Pears
- Mangoes
- Apples
- Kidney beans
- Berries

For fats:

- Avocados
- Full-fat yogurt

- Nuts
- Extra virgin olive oil
- Cheese
- Chia seeds
- Dark chocolate

Intermittent fasting is a frequently studied tool for healthy weight loss. Eating foods such as vegetables, lean proteins, nuts, seeds, and fruits can increase the weight loss benefits of fasting. In order to prevent nutritional deficiencies, healthy eating during a fast is key. Fasting can be combined with popular diets such as the keto diet or a vegetarian diet.

An interesting shift in modern diets is the increased awareness of vegetarianism and veganism. Decreasing the consumption of animal-based foods is beneficial to the environment as farming of animals plays a major role in increasing greenhouse gases. Vegetarians have a lower rate of type 2 diabetes, heart disease, and cancer than those who regularly eat meat as part of their daily diets, according to data indications. Interestingly, vegans do need to supplement the intake of vitamin B12 as their diet is naturally low in it.

The idea that a strict vegetarian diet can impact or even reverse certain diseases is not new. Recent research data indicates that limiting animal products in the diet is beneficial to health in many ways.

A recent study of 198 people put them on a vegetarian diet. Study participants also removed all avocados, nuts, oils, refined sugars, excess salt, processed foods, and fruit juice from their diet. Of the 198 participants, 177 stuck to the plan guidelines entirely and all saw reduced severity of their chronic illness symptoms. A complete reversal of the disease was seen in 22 percent of the participants. The participants were instructed to continue as normal with their prescribed medication during the trial and to become more physically active. Those taking part in the study were also shown how to read food labels properly and given delicious vegetarian meal recipes. While larger studies are required to determine whether only changing over to a vegetarian diet provides any benefit in chronic disease reversal. Whether or not it is a way to reverse disease and increase energy levels, a vegetarian or vegan lifestyle is most certainly a healthier option all round when compared to consuming an excessive amount of animal products. Benefits will also be seen by simple and gradual reduction in the number of animal products you ingest and by increasing the amount of fresh produce you eat. As vegetarianism and the vegan lifestyle become more popular, there are more ready-made vegetarian and vegan products available for purchase. It really is an industry of its own now. Don't assume, however, that because a product has a vegetarian or vegan label on it that it is automatically healthy. No matter what diet you follow while fasting, it is imperative to empower yourself by reading food labels and making yourself aware of exactly what is going into your body (Taylor, n.d.).

Chapter 8:
Best Exercises to Boost Your Libido and Support Your Fast

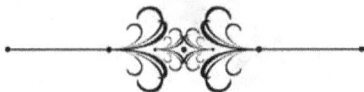

Exercise is an important part of any healthy lifestyle. In intermittent fasting it also helps to boost autophagy and multiply the benefits that we receive from the fasting regime. As women over 50, there are particular considerations when we choose exercise, depending on our fitness starting point and overall health. Exercise does not have to be extremely strenuous and a chore. Instead, it should actually be something that you look forward to and, as such, you should certainly choose a form of exercise that you enjoy and that you can easily incorporate into your life. Increasing your levels of activity can be as simple as choosing the stairs over the elevator or parking that little bit further from the shopping center's entrance. We have phenomenal tools today that can help us to track our activity both in wristwatch form and on our cell phones.

Exercise, in women over 50, can have very specific benefits including increased release of happy hormones, which aid mood stabilization. Certain types of exercises can also help with incontinence and improving flagging libido. Loss of muscle mass is another common occurrence as we age and, this too, can be addressed through proper exercise as well as the types of food we eat after exercise. It is also important for us to understand how best to incorporate exercise with fasting in order to avoid exhausting all of our energy stores.

Exercising While Practicing Intermittent Fasting

Most fasting methods will put you in your fasting window in the morning, which is also the most popular time for exercise. Depending on what your schedule looks like, if you can save your exercise for your eating window, then you should certainly do so. If not, be sure to avoid any extremely strenuous exercises while in your fasting window and if you really want to get the blood flowing use low-impact exercises instead. Always remember to ensure that you are well hydrated when you exercise, especially if it is during your fasting window. While there is evidence that shows that exercising while fasting impacts muscle biochemistry as well as insulin sensitivity, and certain studies have shown that for women with type 2 diabetes or metabolic syndrome, it may be helpful to exercise directly after eating and before food absorption takes place, this evidence is too insufficient to risk damage to our bodies. Exercise while fasting should therefore, always err on the side of low-intensity rather than high-intensity. One of the major concerns for women over 50 is that our muscle mass is already naturally reducing and there is evidence to suggest that when we exercise on an empty stomach, we may start to break down muscle for fuel (Lindberg, 2018).

Low-intensity exercises like walking, jogging, cycling, yoga, Pilates and light cardio are acceptable to do while fasting. Do not exercise for longer than 60 minutes while in your fasting window and if you feel light-headed or unwell, stop immediately. Exercise can be a good distraction from hunger in the initial days of intermittent fasting but it is vital to do exercises that you enjoy so that you are not 'punishing' yourself while also being hungry. This will allow your brain to make positive connections between your activities and encourage you to continue. Interestingly, yoga practitioners prefer to do yoga on an empty stomach as it allows for a lighter feeling and good flow of breath, which is integral to the exercise form. Yoga is a very good choice for women over 50 as it has a mental health boosting effect and it is low-impact on joints. In the same vein as yoga is Pilates which is excellent for strengthening your core muscles. Dance is another great morning/fasting exercise and the high level of coordination and focus required means that you will likely forget about your hunger for the duration. You can attend classes such as Zumba or dance in your own home, whichever you prefer. Walking is a great morning exercise. Take a friend (human or furry) and enjoy early morning fresh air. Making exercise a social activity or one that you do with a pet actually encourages exercise as it is difficult to skip that walk when those mournful canine eyes are imploring you to get your walking shoes on. If you don't live in an area where walking is possible (or safe), treadmills do just as well. In fact, walking on a treadmill which is set to a slight incline burns more fat than walking on a flat surface. Cycling is another great low-impact exercise which can really give a mental boost first thing in the morning.

Boxing, CrossFit, HIIT classes and power lifting are all exercises that should be avoided when exercising in a fasted state.

30-Minute Morning Workout

If you have 30 minutes to spare in the morning and you want to get your blood flowing, we recommend a combination of a 15 minute walk (approximately one mile) followed by 15 minutes of core work, squats, lunges, and pushups. All of the latter exercises can be done in the privacy of your own home. There are many resources available on the internet which you can follow to ensure you get the exercises right.

45-Minute Morning Workout

If your morning is a little more open and you have more time to spare we recommend starting with a jog or brisk walk for approximately 20 to 30 minutes followed by 15 minutes of yoga or bodyweight exercises (Southard, n.d.).

The Importance Of Strength Training After 50

As we age, we start to lose muscle mass and by the age of 50, we can start losing up to 30 percent of our muscle mass. This is not just bad in terms of physical strength but we also then become more prone to injury and illness as we lose our body tone. This natural process can be significantly minimized by taking part in strength training exercises. The knock-on benefits of maintaining and increasing our muscle mass include maintaining our independence—if you retain your strength, you will be able to continue doing things for yourself and you won't have to rely on others as much. As we know, our bone density also decreases as we age and this combined with weaker muscles is a catastrophe waiting to happen.

Unexpected falls are a major cause of death in the elderly every year as breakages take far longer to heal and can allow for infections and all sorts of domino conditions to develop. Weight training also helps to decrease body fat and lower the risk of chronic disease. If you already have chronic disease, weight training can help you to reduce symptoms in cases such as diabetes, depression, and arthritis. As we are also at higher risk for depression as we age, the boost in self-confidence and general mental health wellness that weight training gives us can help to lessen our experience of depression and anxiety. You really only need to allocate about 15 - 30 minutes a day to weight training in order to see all of these benefits. Women over 50 should practice weight training in a very specific way.

10 Weight Training Exercises for Women Over 50

You will need a pair of hand weights (between three and eight pounds) as well as a stability ball. The single-leg moves in these exercises as well as working with the stability ball help to improve balance and coordination which is very important for preventing falls later in life. Perform eight to 12 repetitions for each exercise and rest for 20 to 60 seconds between each type of exercise. Remember to breathe deeply and, as this is all about muscle forming, keep the placement of your limbs correct.

1. **The standard plank:** Lying on the floor, face down, align your elbows directly under your shoulders and ensure that your forearms are flat on the floor. Now, engage your core muscles and lift yourself off the floor. Your body should stay in a straight line. Engage your abdominal muscles and don't let your hips move. Hold this position for 30 seconds. If you experience pain in your lower back, move your knees down onto the ground. This exercise targets your core muscles as well as your shoulder muscles.

2. **The amended push-up:** Start with your hands below your shoulders and your knees behind your hips in a kneeling position. Your back should be angled and long. Tuck your toes under, bend your elbows to lower your chest toward the floor, and tighten your abdominal muscles. Move back upward to the starting position. This exercise

targets your core muscles and arm and shoulder muscles.

3. **The simple squat:** Place your feet hip-distance apart and stand tall. Face your knees, toes, and hips forward. Extend your buttocks outward while bending your knees. Keep your weight distributed on your heels and your knees behind your toes. Rise up and repeat. If you would like to add resistance, you can hold weights while you do this exercise. This exercise targets quads, hamstrings, and glute muscles.

4. **Chest fly with stability ball:** Place your shoulder blades and head on the stability ball while holding the weights close to your chest. The rest of your body should be squared-off against the floor, like a table top, with your feet hip-distance apart. Keeping your palms facing inward, raise the weights together straight up above your chest. With a slight bend in your elbow, turn your lower arms out until your elbows are at chest level. Squeeze your chest and bring hands together again on top. This exercise targets your core muscles, and your back, chest, and glute muscles.

5. **Triceps kick with a stability ball:** Place your chest on the ball, and drape your arms, holding the weights alongside. Your legs should be extended out behind you. Maintain a straight line between your head and your spine. Your arms should be in a 90-degree bend for your starting position. Extend your arms, squeezing your triceps and pressing the weights backward, then release back to the starting point. This exercise targets your triceps and core muscles.

6. **The overhead pass:** Your starting point should be with your feet hip-distance apart. Then create a goal post position with your elbows out to the side and the weights at the side of your head. Keep your abdominal muscles tight. Slowly bring the weights up until your arms are straight and then return to the starting position. This exercise targets biceps, shoulder muscles, and back muscles.

7. **The overhead pull with a stability ball:** With your shoulder blades and head on the ball, and feet hip-distance apart, keep the rest of your body in a table-top position. Pull the weights close to your chest and then raise them straight up with your palms facing inward. Slightly bend your elbow and

then lower your arms behind your head. As you do so, flex your lat muscles and pull arms back into the starting position. This exercise targets your core muscles and back muscles.

8. **Side leg lift with a stability ball:** Your starting position will be kneeling with the ball on your right-hand side, leaning slightly against the wall with your arm draped over it. Stretch your left leg out to the side and keep the right leg bent on the floor. Slowly lift and lower the leg. Then switch to the left side and repeat. This exercise targets leg muscles and core muscles.

9. **Hamstring bridge:** While lying on your back on the floor, bend your knees and keep your feet flat and hip-distance apart. Raise your right leg in the air at a 90-degree angle to the floor. Squeeze your glutes and lift your hips off the floor. Repeat this eight to 12 times and then switch to the other leg and repeat. This exercise targets your glutes, hamstrings, and quads.

10. **The flying dog:** On the floor, kneel on all fours. Stretch an arm out in front of you, drawing in your abdominal muscles as you do and stretch out the opposite leg. Repeat eight to 12 times and then

switch sides. This exercise targets your core muscles and back muscles (Freytag, 2019).

Going South—Improve Your Libido Through Exercise

Some women are known to experience a dip in libido during and after menopause. This is often linked to vaginal dryness, which occurs as a result of hormonal changes as well as changes in muscle structure around this time. The latter is linked to another frustrating and sometimes embarrassing problem for women over 50—incontinence. Both of these issues can cause significant quality of life problems but thankfully, they can be treated in a variety of ways, including the use of exercise and weight training to strengthen the muscles that control these functions. Besides strengthening of muscles, the hormones released when we exercise also help to boost libido and improve overall mood. Some of the exercises that are beneficial in increasing libido include:

- Strength training
- Kegel exercises
- Yoga

- Walking
- Hiking

Strength training is known to be better at boosting libido than cardio exercise as it is better at reducing stress. Stress, of course, is one of the leading causes of reduced libido. The pelvic floor muscles are strengthened by Kegel exercises and this is believed to aid in boosting libido and preventing incontinence. At the gym, machines like the thigh press and the treadmill can help to boost these muscles. Yoga, thanks to its capability to reduce stress and promote relaxation and mindfulness, is thought to be one of the most powerful exercises for boosting your libido. In the same vein, hiking is another excellent method of relaxing, enjoying fresh air and sunshine, and boosting your mood (Guerra, 2019).

While nearly half of older women reported suffering from incontinence, it is not an inevitable part of getting older. It is entirely possible to treat through medication, devices, surgery, and Kegel exercises.

Kegel Exercises

One of the great things about Kegel exercises is that they can be done anywhere. You can do them while you are driving, sitting at your desk, watching television or eating dinner. The key behind Kegel exercises is essentially pretending that you need to urinate and then holding it. You flex and relax the muscles that control the flow of your urine and it is important to ensure that you are flexing the correct muscles to get the best results from your exercises. A good way to identify these muscles is by starting and stopping the flow of urine and being really mindful about exactly which muscles you are using to do so. Once you have managed to identify the location of these muscles and how to send signals from your brain to flex and relax them, you can start doing Kegel exercises. Make sure that you empty your bladder before attempting Kegel exercises. While sitting or lying down, tighten the pelvic floor muscles and hold them for three to five seconds. Then relax the muscles for three to five seconds again. Repeat this 10 times on three occasions during the day (morning, afternoon, and night). While you are doing these exercises be sure to continue breathing deeply and ensure that you are not tightening any other muscles besides the ones you have identified as your pelvic floor muscles. As with anything, it is possible to do too many of these exercises. You should start to experience a difference after about four weeks of practicing Kegel exercises, you should continue to do these exercises otherwise your symptoms will return, but you should not increase the number of times you do them (Medline Plus, n.d.).

New To Exercise? It's Not Too Late

Many of the health issues linked to aging are actually as a result of poor lifestyle choices earlier in life, including low levels of activity. Thankfully, as you consider starting your intermittent fasting journey, it is not too late to change the tide by adding a bit of exercise. If the thought of attempting to cram yourself into anything vaguely resembling lycra and sweating away at the gym while 20-year-olds literally run rings around you, is not your idea of fun, fear not. Exercise does not need to be undertaken at the gym. It doesn't even need to be a formal session at all. It is merely about increasing your activity levels in simple and enjoyable ways. Walking your dog, hiking to bird watch, or even just making healthier choices by taking the stairs or walking to places that are close-by rather than taking your car are all great ways of increasing your activity levels. Aerobic exercises are rather fun, though, and certainly should be a consideration especially if you have a friend who can join you and you can turn it into a morning out for the two of you.

Walking, jogging, dance, and swimming all exercise the large muscles in your body, which aids in strengthening your cardiovascular system. It is, of course, also a great way to burn calories and, hopefully, fat. If you are new to exercise don't try and be a hero on day one! All you will achieve is exhausting yourself, not enjoying the activity and quite likely damaging something. Start with five minutes and slowly work your way up to 20 to 30 minutes of exercise, three or four times a week. Don't exercise every day because your body needs time to heal and grow. A good way to ensure that you are not overdoing your exercise is that you should always be able to have a conversation while exercising. This is called the "talk test" and ensures that you are not pushing yourself to such an extent that you can't breathe properly. If you are so out of breath that you can't talk, that means that you are not getting sufficient oxygen into your system and that is bad news.

If you choose a form of exercise that you enjoy, you will be far more likely to continue to do it and look forward to it (Davis, 2007).

Best Workout Foods

Certain foods will support your workout as well as the healing and growth of muscles better than others. Try to get into the habit of choosing your workout based on the macronutrients you consumed either the day before your workout or that you plan to consume after your workout. Strength building exercises generally require higher levels of carbohydrates on the day of the workout while cardio exercises do better with carbohydrates having been consumed the day before. We have discussed the importance of trying to time your workouts so that it falls within your eating window. It is also quite important to plan what you are going to eat after your workout based on the type of exercise you have done. For instance, if you do weight training and muscle building exercise, you definitely want to take in more protein in your post-workout meal. Ideally you should follow any strength training exercise with a meal that contains carbohydrates and about 20 grams of protein within half an hour of your workout ending. This will take some planning but it is absolutely possible to accomplish (Lindberg, 2018). One of the best ways to structure your eating in the most healthy way across the board is to use the Healthy Eating Plate format. The Healthy Eating Plate is an infographic, created by Harvard School of Public Health. It details how much of each type of food should be eaten in a day. To begin with, vegetables and fruits should take up half of your plate. It's better if vegetables make up more of this half as some fruits are high in sugar. Potatoes are not considered vegetables in this context, and keep in mind that potatoes have a negative impact on blood sugar. Include as many different types of vegetables and colors of fruit as possible.

The second half of the plate is split in two. Half of that (a quarter of the plate) should be filled with whole grains or intact grains such as whole grain bread, pasta, or brown rice. Refined grains like white bread and rice should be limited as they negatively impact blood sugar. The last quarter of the plate is for a healthy protein such as fish, beans, or nuts. Cheese and red meat should be limited and processed meats, bacon, and cold cuts, should be avoided completely. Where beverages are concerned the guide recommends tea, water, or coffee with as little sugar and milk as possible. Any dairy drinks should be limited to two servings per day, and unsweetened fruit juice should be kept at one glass a day. Cut out carbonated, sugary drinks completely. Opt for healthy oils such as peanut, olive, sunflower, corn, or canola oil as salad dressings and when cooking. Limit butter consumption, and avoid trans fats completely. If you haven't caught on yet, the main focus of this guide is that quality is (usually) more important than quantity. How much carbohydrates you have on your plate is less important than the quality of carbohydrates. Legume and vegetable sources of carbohydrates are a much better choice than potatoes. Like fasting, the Healthy Eating Plate doesn't dictate exact quantities or calorie counts but we can use the plate as a guide to ensure we are eating a balanced diet (The Nutrition Source, n.d.).

Chapter 9:
Real Life Stories From Women in Your Shoes

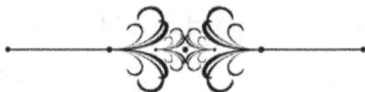

There is no better proof of a regime's efficacy than the changes it has made in the lives of real people. Reading about studies and statistics is all very reassuring but there is really no better assurance and inspiration than knowing that someone just like you has already overcome their challenges and seen success using intermittent fasting. We have collected five real-life stories from ordinary women who achieved extraordinary results with intermittent fasting. Their stories are in their own words and from their personal perspective.

I Lost 25 Pounds for My Daughter's Wedding

In June last year, I received the most amazing news from my daughter Tahlia. She had just become engaged to her long-time boyfriend, Peter, and we had to start planning a wedding. While the engagement came as no surprise as the two had been in a serious relationship for some time, their timeline was a little more frightening. They wanted to be married in October. While four months is probably not an impossible time frame to plan a wedding in, it certainly made me anxious for another reason. Having recently experienced menopause, I had slowly picked up weight, until, eventually, as I described to my husband, "I feel like a pork sausage!"—and that wasn't my way of describing what I wanted for my next snack either. I really felt terrible about myself. My husband was amazingly supportive. He said all the right things about how he thought I was beautiful no matter what I weighed, but I couldn't help feeling down every time I looked in the mirror. I took no joy in trying on new outfits anymore and my daughter and I hadn't gone on one of our mom-and-daughter shopping trips in ages.

While I had never been the "skinny girl," I had never been at the weight I was at that time either. I needed to lose at least 25 pounds before my daughter's wedding or my new apple-shape would be recorded in photographs for all of eternity. My grandchildren would look at their mother's wedding album and exclaim, "Oh look at Grandma!" Within a week, we had planned Tahlia and Peter's engagement party and the Saturday saw me arriving late to my own daughter's event because my husband had to drag me out of the house after I had discarded the umpteenth outfit on the basis that it made me look like a potato. I eventually relaxed and enjoyed the party but that was a turning point for me. At the party, were friends and family members that I hadn't seen for years. Many of them had never seen me at my current weight and most were kind enough to hide their surprise. One of my cousins attended. She had struggled with her weight her whole life and when I saw her, my jaw almost hit the floor. She looked phenomenal. Alice was a few years older than me and as long as I could remember she had been on every diet known to man. Any fad diet that popped up, Alice tried. She would lose a few pounds but by the time I would see her next she had put the weight back on again. This time, though, something was very different and I had to know what her secret was. When she uttered the words "intermittent fasting," my mind immediately conjured up pictures of monks in the Himalayan mountains refusing themselves food for days on end in penance. Alice laughed and we spent the rest of the evening over a sumptuous plate of food—which I ashamedly picked at and Alice heartily enjoyed—with Alice explaining the concept of intermittent fasting to me.

On the way home, I told my husband my plan. Thankfully, he has always been behind me 100 percent and after we did some more research together on the internet that night, I decided that my intermittent fasting journey would start the next day. In most situations this may seem a little rushed, but let's not forget, I had four months to lose 25 pounds if I wanted to be the slim mother of the bride. I did start slowly because Alice had warned me to. She had tried jumping straight into 16 full hours of fasting in her first week and she had felt terrible. Then, after chatting to a friend who had also started the intermittent fasting lifestyle, she decided to start again, this time slowly working her way up to a 14 hour fast which she felt was best for her. I decided to follow her lead and also started slowly as much as I wanted to leap in head first. In all honesty, I did still struggle with hunger in the beginning. As I had started putting on weight, I had slid into a mild depression and I had been attempting to eat my way out of it. My fasting journey actually made me realize that I had a rather unhealthy relationship with food. Although this was the first time in my life that I had struggled with my weight, I realized that I had always used food as a solace. Fasting helped me to understand that while enjoyment of food is natural, it is there for nourishment and using it as emotional support is a symptom of a larger problem.

The weeks ticked by and although I stumbled occasionally, I was amazed at how I started to feel. I had more energy than I had in years and considering I was planning a wedding; it couldn't have come at a better time. I had never been much of an exerciser but a friend of mine had been bugging me for ages to join her on her morning walks and with my new-found energy, I thought that, at the very least, it would give me an even greater boost in weight loss. It did and I started to see the pounds shedding.

About a month before my daughter's wedding, though, just when I thought all was on track, I hit a wall. The weight stopped moving and, although at this point I had already lost a significant amount, I still wasn't exactly where I wanted to be. I called Alice and she suggested extending my fast by just one hour. I did this and, as we near the big day I hit my goal!

It was indescribable to be able to be back to the weight I wanted to be but the feeling of achievement was more than that. For much of my adult life, I had based my health on luck but now I realized that, in order to live a happy and long life, I was going to have to put a little effort in and I was fine with that. The rewards were more than worth it.

Four months after I made that decision, I stood next to my beautiful daughter as she entered into a new phase of her life. She, of course, was the princess of the day but I was proud to stand next to her and she was proud of me. Although she was pleased with my weight loss, she later told me that it had nothing to do with how proud she felt. She confessed that I had inspired her and that she now knew that women could be strong, fit and beautiful their entire lives if they just made the right choices and stuck to them. On that day, I could have chosen to stop my intermittent fasting journey right there. I had achieved my goal, after all, but I didn't. I chose to make intermittent fasting a permanent part of my lifestyle because regardless of what I weighed, I had seen real and phenomenal benefits in so many other areas and I never wanted to go back to where I had been before I started.

Mandy, 55, Self-Employed Accountant

I Conquered My Autoimmune Dysfunctions With Intermittent Fasting

Although I had been living with two autoimmune diseases from the age of 40 when I was diagnosed, when menopause hit me at the age of 52, I really started going downhill. Although I should have still had at least another 10 years as a teacher—a job I loved with all of my heart—my conditions had forced me to resign. The ulcerative colitis which I had been able to manage with medication and diet for years suddenly exploded out of control during my menopause.

Nothing my doctor tried helped and eventually I had to admit that having to run to the toilet every half an hour was not conducive to doing my job well. It broke my heart but I also just didn't have the energy the kids needed from me anymore. Around the same time my colitis had been diagnosed, I had also been diagnosed with lupus, another autoimmune disorder. That diagnosis had been a little more frightening as lupus can be deadly. As with the colitis, though, I had been blessed to be able to keep the symptoms under control with medication and good nutrition. After my menopause started, though, I felt like I was living in someone else's body. My lupus medication stopped working too and my hands became stiff and painful. I had cried as I walked out of the school that I had taught at for so many years. Some of those tears were for my lost career, but most were the result of sheer terror. I felt like my body was killing itself and I had absolutely no control over what happened anymore.

A week after my resignation, I found myself seated on my bathroom floor in floods of tears with hands that were so stiff I could barely move my fingers. I didn't even have the energy to get back up and move to the couch. My sister found me there later. I'd fallen asleep on the bathroom floor. Of course, at first, she freaked out thinking I had collapsed, after she had established that I was just having a physical and emotional meltdown she sat next to me on the floor for what seemed like hours. My sister is a fixer. She has tried for years to help me find a solution to my symptoms and she wasn't about to give up even though I was ready to.

"I came across this blog the other day." She said quite out of the blue. I grunted in response. Without thinking, she tried to pass her phone to me so that I could read it too but quickly realized my hands were not in a phone-gripping state. She read it to me. The blog was by a woman called Marion, who had opened a very special Bed and Breakfast after an experience that had changed her life. She had been morbidly obese and her doctors had basically told her that if she didn't make big changes soon, she was going to die. In her blog, she explained how she had started intermittent fasting and it had saved her life. There was a huge amount of information on fasting on her blog and the interesting part was that it showed major benefits for people with autoimmune disorders. After this life-changing experience she had opened her Bed and Breakfast which she fondly referred to as a Bed and No-Breakfast Retreat. People booked into the venue for weeks at a time and she helped them to get started on their intermittent fasting journey.

The next day, my sister called to tell me that she had booked me into the fasting retreat. I argued with her but had little energy to do so, and, in the end, she won and I relented. I figured that I had tried everything else and I really had nothing to lose. I would try this intermittent fasting thing and if it worked, great, if it didn't, it was just another thing I could cross off my list. Although I went into fasting with a "let's see" attitude, I really hoped that it would work. I could only think that the next option would be medication which would probably have more side effects than anything else. Amazingly, although I have always been a really logical person and not one to jump to conclusion, this downward spiral in my health really had me seeing the worst case scenario and I often found myself in tears at the thought of losing my battle and leaving my family alone.

My first few days at the retreat were interesting. Marion was a firecracker and immediately jumped into action. She explained how fasting could help to heal the microbiota in my gut which, in part, were responsible for the unreliable signals that my autoimmune system was getting. She also explained how fasting could reduce inflammation and then told me about the real kicker—autophagy. The idea that I could use my own body's processes to rebuild new and undamaged cells, essentially overhauling my immune system was exciting. Before the fasting actually started, I had to address my diet and own up to the fact that my eating habits, although generally not the worst, were starting to slowly unravel the sicker I got. Mentally, I had got to the point where I had actually given up and the processed foods that I was putting into my body as comfort, were only making my conditions worse. We started with the intermittent fasting slowly and then worked our way up to 16 hours. Within a week, my trips to the toilet had slowed to two a day. I was officially impressed. I also felt the stiffness in my hand starting to relax slightly. Every day, I felt a little better. By the second week, I was using the onsite gym, something I thought I would never have the energy for. By my third and final week at the Marion's retreat, my hands were no longer stiff at all and I felt better than I had in my entire life, if I was honest.

Marion prepared me well for my return home so that I could continue my fasting journey there, although honestly with the benefits I was already seeing, you couldn't have force fed me in my fasting window if you tried. Within three months of my return home I felt like a completely different person. My toilet habits were normal. The stiffness in my joints was gone. My sister could not believe her eyes and, of course, the 'fixer' in her was deeply satisfied.

A year later, I called the school that I had resigned from and asked if they had any open posts. They welcomed me back with open arms and I was able to continue doing the job I loved. I still practice intermittent fasting to this day and my doctors are pretty astonished at my recovery. I now advocate for the use of intermittent fasting as an accompanying therapy in all of the autoimmune disease support groups I belong to. I realize that not everyone will have the same results that I did but what I think intermittent fasting does is give you back your power. Those who have never suffered from an autoimmune disease will not understand the devastation of knowing that your own immune system, that is supposed to protect you, is making you sick. It makes you feel completely powerless. Fasting gave me, not just my health and career back, but also the feeling that I am in control of my own body.

Wendy, 53, Teacher

I Thought I Had Dementia

Menopause arrived rather late for me but when it did I knew it was there. I was 55 by the time I had my first inkling that menopause was making itself known in my life but, honestly, I was so busy that I didn't take much notice. My career has always been extremely important to me. I'm a research scientist for a large university and my work is detailed and takes a lot of focus. This had never been a problem for me because, even throughout my pregnancies with my children, my cognitive abilities had always been sharp and highly honed. It was something I took great pride in. Which is probably why when I suddenly started to forget things, it hit me like a ton of bricks. I had expected some side effects from menopause and the hot flashes, night sweats, and occasional constipation was manageable for me. I remember thinking that this menopause thing is not that difficult. Then I got to work one morning, sat down at my lab bench as I always did, pulled out my laptop to start funneling some data from the day before, and I couldn't remember my password. It was the same password I had used for the last five years (terrible e-security, I know!), but, for the life of me, at that moment I couldn't tell you what it was.

When I mentioned it to my partner that night, he suggested that maybe I just needed a bit of a break. I had been feeling tired but I was used to working long hours. I relented as I felt that it couldn't hurt to take a few days off. I could always do some work from home if I got bored. I applied for a two-week leave the next day and my surprised boss agreed, considering I had never taken anything more than a day or two of leave before that. I worked a full day, still feeling like I was looking through a fog. I had written my password in my diary in case I forgot it again, but I continued to feel confused and out of sorts. That afternoon as I left I said goodbye to my boss and said I'd see him the next day. He looked at me strangely asking if I had changed my mind about my leave. Embarrassed, I made a joke of having forgotten. I took my laptop with me but by the time I got home and pulled into my driveway, I couldn't find it anywhere. I drove back to the university and to my horror, found my laptop smashed in the parking lot. I had put it on top of my car to unlock my door and forgotten it there. Driving away, it had slipped off and smashed everywhere. My boss came out to find me, in tears, picking up pieces of my laptop off the floor. Although he was really lovely about it, telling me not to worry and that accidents happen, I was devastated. I knew the laptop could be replaced but I had never done anything like that before. Not even at my busiest or most distracted had I forgotten something like that. I could only hope that taking leave would help.

My partner worked from home so I had some company. I had no idea how to do this "time off" thing, having been a workaholic my entire life. I did some crafts, and then tried to read a book. I say 'tried' because I had eventually had to give up. By the time I got to the end of the second chapter, I could no longer remember what had happened in the first. I couldn't focus. I kept on wondering where all of these new characters were coming from only to page back and realize they had been introduced on the second page of the book. With a shaking hand, I closed the book and placed it on my bedside table.

"I'm going for a run." I burst into my partner's study, completely forgetting that he had told me just five minutes before that he was starting a Skype call with a client. Now the client also knew that I was going for a run. I was mortified. He laughed about it later but his concern was evident. He didn't care that I had interrupted his call, he was really worried that I was suddenly unable to remember information from just minutes before. As I started my jog, I thought about my mom who had died years before. She had developed dementia and with a sick feeling that was so profound that I stopped running, I wondered if I was developing the same dreaded disease. Surely I was too young for that? I know that, for many people, the level of forgetfulness I was experiencing would be nothing out of the ordinary. We bombard our brains with information and often overload them and as a result, we forget things. That wasn't me, though, I had never experienced this feeling and it was terrifying. My job depended on my cognitive ability. If I couldn't recall or process information, my career was over. For most, early retirement would not be the worst thing in the world but I had built my identity around my work and the value that I felt it added to the world. While this may sound rather emotionally unhealthy, I was able to recognize that I wouldn't be able to do my job forever but I wasn't quite ready to throw the towel in. I really felt that I had a lot more to give the world of research.

By the end of my two-week vacation at home, I was all but useless to myself and anyone else, or at least that is how I felt. I had no choice but to call my boss and, in tears, (after forgetting his name), tell him that I would have to take an extended leave of absence from work. I had to get a doctor's opinion as I was now entirely convinced that I was developing dementia.

24-hours later I sat in my doctor's office expecting him to tell me the worst news of my life. I had explained my symptoms—the forgetfulness, the feeling of continuously thinking through a fog—and he didn't look at all concerned. In fact, he had a small smile on his face when he said to me, "You know you are in menopause, right?"

I stopped myself from biting off his head as I explained that although I was well aware that I was in menopause, I had experienced very few side effects and surely, this devastating loss of cognitive function could not be related to that? If I had been embarrassed at my forgetfulness it had been nothing compared to the mortification I experienced when I realized that, if I had just done some research (which should have been my natural reaction) I would have realized that memory fog, forgetfulness, and a loss of cognitive function are all very common side effects of menopause. He went on to explain that hormones are extremely powerful and as my body sorted out its new levels, things like this were going to happen. He then told me that I was actually lucky that I hadn't experienced most of the other symptoms that other women do. Sadly, this symptom, for me, was the last one I needed. We discussed my options and decided that hormone replacement therapy was not the way to go for me. I had a history of heart disease in my family and considering this was my only symptom, such a treatment would be overkill. The reason I enjoyed going to this doctor was because he wasn't one to push medication at any opportunity and what he suggested next confirmed that he hadn't changed his stance on that. "Try intermittent fasting for a month or so and see how you feel."

I wrote down everything he told me and then went home feeling slightly better. At least I had a plan. It did sound a bit odd that changing the way I eat could have such a huge impact on my brain but he was a doctor, after all, so I decided to give it a try. My first day of intermittent fasting was a bit of a fail as I forgot that I was supposed to be fasting and prepared a sumptuous breakfast for my partner and me. He said nothing and we ate and enjoyed our breakfast. After we were finished he suggested that I put up some notes around the kitchen to remind me that I was supposed to be fasting. Day two became day one and the notes worked. Being at home with little to occupy me did make the first few days more difficult than they needed to be but I managed to press through. If nothing else, I could prove to my doctor that this was not caused by hormones and he would be forced to do further testing. By week two, I was starting to feel more like my old self. My partner noticed that it was now possible to have conversations with me again because I wasn't continuously forgetting what we were talking about and having to blurt things out before I forgot what I had wanted to say. Slowly and in daily increments the fog lifted. Never in my life had I been so pleased to be proved wrong. Once I had regained my cognitive abilities, I noticed other changes. I had lost a bit of the extra weight I had gained, which was an added bonus, and my skin looked clearer.

I was able to return to work a month after I had taken an extended leave of absence and I could not have been happier. My work was actually better than it had ever been and our research department would go on to win several grants based on the work I did in those months after returning. Even though my menopause is now a thing of the past and I could probably go back to eating normally and not experience the same memory issues, I decided to continue with intermittent fasting. I felt better than I ever had in my life and there was no way I was letting go of that feeling.

Samantha, 57, Research Scientist

Fasting Cured My Early-Onset Arthritis

I was not new to intermittent fasting by any means. It had been something that my family had sworn by for decades, before it was as popular as it is today. My mom had used intermittent fasting to lose her post-baby weight and her menopausal weight and my dad had been the only one in his family to avoid developing heart disease, which he put down to a lifetime of fasting. Mealtimes in my house growing up were pretty much structured around fasting so it was very much a lifestyle for us and not just a weight loss method. We understood all of the related benefits before it was so hugely popular. As you grow up, though, you often start to believe that you know better and the way I managed my health was no different.

I had followed the regime in my 20s and 30s but when I had children, I hadn't continued and never found my way back to it. It was still something that I recommended to others but I was feeling in good health, my weight was good and I didn't see any reason to get back into fasting at that time in my life. That was until I woke up one morning at age 50, with an incredible pain in my shoulder. At first I thought I had just overdone my training session the day before. I decided to rest for a few days, took some anti inflammatories, and hoped for the best. The medication helped while I was taking it but I couldn't stay on it for too long and, as a freelance writer, the grogginess from the tablets, paired with the pain in my shoulder when I typed on my computer, were becoming serious problems. Then I started to feel stiffness in my fingers and a burning sensation in my joints. My knees were painful when I got up in the morning and I struggled to walk. It was time to go to the doctor. His diagnosis threw me for a loop. I had arthritis. I was stunned. Surely I was far too young for arthritis. It happens, my doctor explains, early-onset arthritis is not uncommon. He prescribed medication and some dietary changes. I ate more oily fish, cruciferous vegetables and had fruit-filled smoothies as often as I could. This all helped slightly but I still couldn't carry on with my normal exercise routine and had to change to lower impact exercises, which I didn't really enjoy as much. One Sunday afternoon, I was sitting at my mother's house for a family lunch bemoaning my fate and the fact that I had to shorten my working hours as, after a few hours I just couldn't type anymore. My father asked me if I had forgotten about fasting. In annoyance, I snapped at him that I couldn't take my medication if I wasn't eating. In his usual calm demeanor, he reminded me of all of the benefits that fasting holds. Things started to fall into place in my mind and later on I did some research into the impact of fasting on inflammation. I decided to give it a try. After all, I couldn't make it any worse. I worked out a plan to take my medication on schedule during my eating window and I got back into fasting. After not having fasted for almost 20 years, it was a bit of a struggle to get back into it. The pain that I was in made my grumpy and being hungry didn't help so I think that in those first few days, those around me wished they could be somewhere else. To be honest, I wished that I could be in someone else's body too.

I took a leap and cut meat out of my diet too. In some of the resources I read, red meat was shown to have an inflammatory effect on those suffering with arthritis. I became a pescatarian feeling that the omega-3 from fish could still have a positive impact. Slowly but surely, I started to feel better. I felt the impact in my fingers first. They felt looser and I could type for longer. Then one morning I got out of bed and the shot of pain in my shoulder that had become my constant companion was gone.

As the days went on, my stiffness and pain incrementally subsided. I spoke to my doctor about weaning off my medication and he agreed. Three months after I had been diagnosed with arthritis, I was symptom free and able to return to my normal exercise regime. I realize now that if I had just continued with an intermittent fasting lifestyle after having my children, I probably never would have had to go through this. Lesson learned!

Maria, 52, Homemaker

Bonus Chapter:
Intermittent Fasting Kickstart

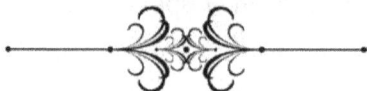

As a kickstart to your intermittent fasting journey we have put together a three-day plan to ease you into your journey.

We have included some ideas for exercises as well as meal ideas. We will ease you into a 16-hour fast by starting at 12 hours and increasing by two hours every day. If you wish to stretch out further than that, you can easily do so.

Day One

Our Message

Welcome to the first day of your intermittent fasting journey. You are about to start retraining your body to do what it was always meant to. We can't promise it is going to be easy, but we can definitely promise you that it will be worth it. Today is a momentous day as it marks the start of a journey that will not only have an impact on your body in the short term but also in the long term. The longer you are able to keep up your intermittent fasting, the longer you will see results. Do your best to start today with a sense of positivity. If you wake up with a sense of dread, don't take that with you into the rest of the day, make sure you sort it out right away.

Suggested Eating Window

For your first day of fasting, we recommend that you set your eating window from 8 a.m. to 8 p.m. In other words you can have your first meal at 10 a.m. but you must have had your last meal by 8 p.m. You will then fast from 8 p.m.

Suggested Meals

As you have only just started your fasting journey, you will be using today's meals to prepare yourself for your coming fasting window. To do this, you will want to eat as many fruit and vegetables as possible and provide yourself with the macronutrients that you will need for exercise and for the autophagy process.

10 a.m. meal

Smoothies are an excellent way to break your fast. They are easy on your stomach and it's also a great way to pack your nutrients in. When making smoothies try not to only include fruits as this can make your smoothie extremely sweet and could push your blood sugar up too high. Try mixing fruits and vegetables together and include good fats like avocado, chia seeds, and flaxseed.

The following fruit and vegetable combinations go really well together:

- carrot and orange
- spinach and orange
- apple and cucumber
- apricots and sweet potato

- spinach and mango
- carrot and green apple
- asparagus and strawberry

The following is our suggestion for your smoothie of the day:

Option 1: Green Ginger Smoothie

- 1-inch piece of ginger
- 1 cup coconut water
- 1 handful baby kale leaves
- 1 cup frozen mango chunks
- 1 handful baby spinach leaves

Whizz all the ingredients up in the food processor, adding small amounts of coconut water until you reach your preferred consistency. This makes two servings and freezes really well, so you can drink one serving and freeze the other for another day. These are great for summer as you can take them out the freezer an hour or two before you want to drink them and then you will have an iced smoothie to cool you down in the summer heat.

Option 2: Nutritious Cornmeal Biscuits

Prepare a batch of these beforehand to enjoy as a nutritious meal to break your fast or as a snack during your eating window.

- 2 oz each of raisins, pine nuts, walnuts, almonds, and dried fig
- 9 oz cornmeal
- extra virgin olive oil
- 1 1/2 tbsp sugar
- salt and pepper
- hot water

Preheat the oven to 300 °F. Place the cornmeal into a bowl and form a well in the middle into which you pour a few tablespoons of oil. Soak the raisins, then pat dry and finely chop the other ingredients. Pour the chopped ingredients and raisins into the well with the sugar and a pinch of salt and pepper. Combine well and add water to form a moist but malleable consistency. Form balls with the mixture and flatten with a fork. Bake for half an hour.

12 p.m. meal

For lunch you really want to keep it light while still nourishing and filling enough to keep you going until dinner. In this suggested dip, we include delicious, creamy avocado which is an excellent source of good fat, as well as black beans and cheese for that protein kick. Eat the dip either as a spread on whole wheat toast or with vegetable fingers like carrots and celery for dipping. Healthy and scrumptious!

Option 1: Warm Avo And Bean Dip

- 1 avocado (peeled, pitted and mashed)
- 15-oz can black beans
- 1 clove garlic
- 1 tbsp lime juice
- ⅓ cup shredded cheddar cheese

Mix all ingredients in a bowl and microwave on high until the cheese melts. You can also have this dip cold and leave the cheese out. If you need a little more seasoning, add some sea salt after tasting.

Option 2: Tuscan Salad

- sliced cucumber
- cubed tomatoes

- thinly sliced green onion
- stale Tuscan bread
- red wine vinegar
- fresh basil leaves
- extra virgin olive oil

Soak the bread, squeeze out the water and then let it sit in the fridge for half an hour. In a large bowl, place the other salad ingredients and dress with olive oil, vinegar, and salt. Add the bread and then mix gently to coat. Allow to sit for about half an hour before serving.

7:30 p.m. meal

This is going to be the meal that is going to take you through your first fasting window so it needs to be protein-rich and packed with nutrients. Salmon is a phenomenal source of omega-3 and green leafy vegetables are the superstars of the nutrient rankings.

Option 1: Salmon, Spinach, and Tomato Bake

- 4 pieces of salmon
- 1 cup sliced mushrooms
- 2 cups fresh spinach
- 1 chopped tomato

Preheat the oven to 375 °F. Prepare an oven dish by spraying with nonstick spray. Place fish pieces skin-side down in the dish. Mix all the other ingredients and spoon over the fish pieces. Bake for approximately 25 minutes or until the fish flakes with a fork.

Option 2: White Wine Snapper

- 35 oz snapper
- 5 oz tomatoes
- 7 oz black olives
- ¾ cup white wine
- pepper
- extra virgin olive oil

Preheat the oven to 320 °F. Wash and dry the fish and arrange in a greased casserole dish. Scatter the tomatoes, olives and pepper over the fish and bake for 30 minutes, adding the white wine at the 15-minute mark.

Suggested Routine

Morning Routine

As part of your morning routine, you may want to include some light cardio exercise such as 15 minutes of walking, jogging, swimming, or yoga.

Evening Routine

As part of your evening routine try to include 10 minutes of meditation with essential oils that are good for relaxation like lavender and rosemary.

Day Two

Our Message

Only your second day of fasting will directly follow the first day so that you experience a successive eating and fasting windows to start the process. Thereafter, it is advisable to have a break day between fasting. On your second day, you are going to experience your first fasting window. You are starting with a 12-hour fast to make things easier for you. Even if this first fasting window feels really easy for you, we don't advise you to push it further in terms of hours. The importance of building up your fasting window is not entirely for you to consciously feel that you are capable, it is also so that your body is able to slowly adjust so that you experience fewer side effects.

Today you will shorten your eating window by two hours and, therefore, increase your fasting window by two hours.

Suggested Eating Window

For your second day of fasting, we recommend that you set your eating window from 10 a.m. to 8 p.m. In other words you can have your first meal at 10 a.m.

but you must have had your last meal by 8 p.m. You will then fast from 8 p.m. onward.

Suggested Meals

For day two we will still include three meals but from day three we will decrease this to two meals which should be your set number going forward.

10 a.m. meal

We are huge proponents of the power of the smoothie but another highly effective and nutritious way to break your fast is bone broth. An ideal way of making bone broth is in a large quantity and then freezing it in individual portions to use later. This way you always have a highly nutritious and light meal at hand, with which to break your fast.

Option 1: Beef Bone Broth

- 5 lb beef marrow bones
- 20 cups of water
- 2 bay leaves
- 2 tbsp cider vinegar
- Vegetables and herbs of your choice (carrots, onions, garlic, celery, garlic, parsley etc.)

Preheat the oven to 400 °F. Wash and pat dry the bones being careful to retain the marrow. Arrange the bones on a baking tray and bake until browned. This usually takes about 30 minutes. Once the bones are browned, put them into a large pot with the water, vinegar, vegetables, and bay leaves. Cook for about 24 hours on a low temperature, occasionally skimming anything that has floated to the top. When cooked, strain the broth to remove any solids and then allow the broth to cool so that any fat floats to the top. You can then scoop this solidified fat off the top. Once cooled, freeze in meal-sized portions.

Option 2: Vegetable Broth

Follow the directions for bone broth above but include only vegetables and plenty of nutritious herbs.

12 a.m. meal

Today we recommend some weight training exercises so we are including a high-protein lunch. As far as animal proteins go, chicken is about the healthiest as it is very low in fat, especially if you remove the skin or go for an already skinned and deboned fillet as we use in this recipe.

Option 1: Chicken Salad Sandwich

- 1 deboned chicken breast
- ¼ tsp garlic salt
- 2 tbsp mayonnaise
- 1 tsp finely chopped celery

Steam chicken breast for about 20-30 minutes depending on size. Allow to cool. Shred or cube the meat as soon as it is cool enough to touch as it will cool quicker. When completely cooled, add garlic salt, mayonnaise, and celery. Serve in whole-wheat bread as a sandwich or in a whole-wheat wrap.

Option 2: Herbed Pumpkin

- 35 oz pumpkin flesh
- fresh sage
- fresh rosemary
- honey to taste
- salt to taste

Preheat the oven to 300 °F. Place the cut up pumpkin onto a baking sheet and sprinkle with sage, rosemary, honey and salt. Bake for half an hour until the pumpkin is tender.

7.30 p.m. meal

Where possible, we recommend avoiding animal proteins and instead, learning to enjoy plant-based proteins, which have far more long-term health benefits.

Option 1: Lentil Spaghetti Bolognese

- 1 can lentils
- 15 mushrooms
- 1 can chopped tomatoes
- 3 cups zucchini
- 4 cloves garlic
- 1 onion
- 1 tbsp olive oil
- 1 leek
- Fresh thyme and marjoram to taste
- 9 ½ oz spaghetti
- shaved parmesan (for serving)

In a large frying pan, heat the olive oil over a medium heat and saute the onion until translucent. Add the leek, lentils, garlic, herbs, and mushrooms and fry together for about five minutes. Add the tomatoes and zucchini and season to taste. Simmer for above five minutes until the zucchini is cooked.

While your sauce is cooking, add your spaghetti to a large pot of salted boiling water and cook for about 10 minutes or until al dente. Serve with shaved parmesan.

Option 2: Bean Pesto Linguine

- 11 oz shelled fava beans
- 11 oz linguine
- 1 clove of garlic
- ½ cup of extra virgin olive oil
- fresh mint

In a food processor, place the fava beans and the garlic with a few leaves of mint and some olive oil. Whizz it up until you reach a pesto texture. In the meantime, cook your pasta in salted boiling water until al dente. Retain some of the cooking water to thin out your sauce if it is too thick. Toss the pasta in the fava bean pesto and when you have achieved your desired consistency, serve sprinkled with a few leaves of mint.

Suggested Routine

Morning Routine

Spend some time reflecting on your goals. What do you want to achieve with your fasting journey? Ensure that you are really specific about what you want to achieve. If your goal is weight loss, exactly how much weight do you want to lose and by what date. Also ensure that your goal is realistic. If you slowly gained 10 pounds over the course of a year, is it really realistic to expect to lose it over the course of two weeks? Setting your goals is a mix between being kind to yourself and pushing yourself enough to achieve what you want to.

Afternoon Routine

Today we recommend some weight training exercises to start building your muscles and creating that strong body you want. You can use the exercises that we explained to you earlier in the book. The protein-rich meal that you eat at lunch time will help you to grow your muscles and heal after exercise. Remember to stay hydrated.

Day Three

Our Message

You have made it to day three! By now you should start getting over any of the side effects you might have experienced, such as headaches and you are going to move up to 16 hours of fasting today. Try to maintain a 16-hour fast for the next few days and see how you feel. If necessary you can drop back down to 14 hours and go from there.

Suggested Eating Window

For your third day of fasting, we recommend that you set your eating window from 12 a.m. to 8 p.m. In other words you can have your first meal at 12 a.m. but you must have had your last meal by 8 p.m. You will then fast from 8 p.m. onward.

Suggested Meals

Today you will have your first meal at 12 p.m. While it is not absolutely necessary that you only stick to two meals, you do want to watch your calorie intake, only because it is very easy to overeat when you know that your eating time is now restricted. If you did your preparation and you know how many calories you usually eat outside of fasting, then you should be able to track your meals just for a few days to make sure you aren't binging for the sake of it.

12 p.m. meal

As you have now fasted for an extended period, you will want to be careful about breaking your fast. A smoothie or bone broth would be a great way to nutritiously break your fast. Salads with protein and good fats are another good way to get your nutrients in while still ensuring that your meal is light enough not to leave you feeling ill.

Option 1: Sardine and Mushroom Salad

- 4 sardines
- 12 oz mushrooms
- 1 cup baby spinach
- 6 oz gorgonzola cheese
- 8 tbsp of a vinaigrette of your choice

In a zip lock bag, add your cleaned and washed sardines as well as three tablespoons of the vinaigrette of your choice. Seal the bag and toss until the fish is completely coated. In a large salad bowl, add sliced mushrooms and five tablespoons of your vinaigrette, toss to coat. Add the spinach leaves on top of the mushrooms but don't toss. Heat a frying pan over medium heat and flash fry the sardines for a few minutes then roughly slice. Toss spinach and mushrooms, top with sliced sardines and then garnish with cheese.

Option 2: Hummus

- 2 tbsp tahini paste
- juice of one lemon
- 7 oz dried chickpeas
- 2 cloves of garlic
- fresh parsley
- paprika
- 2 tbsp extra virgin olive oil

Soak the chickpeas overnight and then boil until soft ensuring that you retain some of the cooking liquid. When cooled, blend in a food processor until creamy. Add the juice of the lemon and two tablespoons of cooking liquid. Blend in the processor. Add the garlic, a little salt, and tahini and blend. Scoop out into a bowl, add oil and sprinkle with paprika and fresh parsley. Eat on whole wheat bread as a spread or with pieces of vegetable as a dip.

7.30 p.m. meal

Curry is an extremely nutritious meal and it contains ingredients such as turmeric, garlic, and ginger which are known natural anti-inflammatories. Chickpeas are a great source of continuous energy and will keep you feeling fuller for longer.

Option 1: Chickpea Curry

- 16 oz can of chickpeas
- 1 tsp fresh ginger
- 2 tsp curry powder
- 1 tsp cumin powder
- 1 tsp cilantro powder
- 1 tsp turmeric powder
- 5 cloves of garlic
- 1 can chopped tomatoes
- 3 tbsp olive oil
- water for cooking
- 1 onion

Heat a saucepan over a medium heat with the olive oil. Fry onions for three minutes until translucent. Add spices, ginger, and garlic and allow to cook together for about a minute. Add the chickpeas and about a tablespoon of water. Stir while cooking for about a minute. Add the tinned tomatoes and cook for five minutes, occasionally stirring gently so that it doesn't stick to the pan. If necessary add tablespoons of water as you go to keep it from sticking. Serve with your choice of carbohydrate as a side or as is.

Option 2: Mushroom Polenta

- 3 ½ oz mushrooms
- 3 oz polenta
- fresh parsley
- salt
- 2 tbsp extra virgin olive oil

Cook polenta and set aside. In a medium pan, heat some oil and cook the mushroom with a small amount of water until tender. Add the parsley and stir for a few seconds. Remove from heat and top polenta with mushroom mix.

Suggested Routine

You have learned the science behind what is happening in your body as you fast. This is a good thing to focus on when you experience hunger. Close your eyes and think about the amazing processes that are happening in your body right now. Your cells are renewing themselves and every minute that you stay on your fast, you get healthier. If that is not worth a few hours of a rumbling tummy, then I don't know what is! Remember to drink water when you are really feeling the pinch and consider herbal teas with no additives. The process of making the tea really helps to distract you.

Afternoon Routine

Today we recommend a mix of cardio and weight training. You can choose whether you do them directly after one another or if you give yourself a break between. Always ensure that you can maintain the talk test and keep yourself hydrated. If at any time you feel ill or light-headed, take a break until you feel better.

Evening Routine

Yoga is a great evening exercise as it is relaxing and helps focus your mindfulness. Try doing a few yoga stances about an hour before bed and then meditate for 10 minutes to really calm yourself. Sleep is when your body has the chance to repair itself and take advantage of additional blood flow to areas besides your muscles. If you are struggling to sleep, use an essential oil burner next to your bed and be sure to switch off any electronic devices at least an hour before sleeping.

The Road Ahead

You have successfully completed your first three days of fasting. Give yourself a pat on the back and then sit down to make some decisions. You will need to continue with a 16-hour fast for a few days to really get a good idea of whether it is the right length fast for you. Depending on what goals you have set, you may want to readdress them if you decide to go with a shorter fast over a longer one.

Keep in mind that weight loss is far better managed by taking measurements than standing on a scale. When you weigh yourself, you also weigh all of your water weight and your muscle weight so it doesn't give you a reading of the number you want to know—fat weight. The best way to measure fat weight loss is by measuring yourself with a tailor's measuring tape (the material kind). Take your measurements before you start fasting and then again after each week of your fast.

If you are not starting with fasting in order to lose weight but rather to enjoy its many other benefits, you will likely be able to measure your progress simply by how you feel, how much medication you are taking, and your energy levels.

If you have a chronic condition, always ensure that you are undertaking your intermittent fasting journey under the direction of a doctor.

The Power of Essential Oils

For thousands of years, essential oils have been used not only for their aroma but also for their healing qualities and ability to positively impact our emotional and physical wellbeing. Essential oil is actually not an oil, it is a highly concentrated plant component. They can be extracted from various parts of a plant, including leaves, flowers, fruits, woods, and seeds. It can take a huge amount of a plant to produce even a tiny amount of essential oil, which is why some can be very expensive. For example, it takes 4,000 pounds of roses to make one pound of rose oil. Herbs and plants have been used for centuries to treat all sorts of ailments; the use of essential oils is an age-old tradition that has become more popular again in recent years. Essential oils have the ability to trigger emotional, physical, and mental responses. We can use them to sleep and relax, or to focus and wake up. They can be used to improve digestion and clear and brighten skin. Essential oils are far more than just a scent; their healing effects can be broad and far-reaching. Our ancestors understood that mother nature has given us a wide array of plant extracts with powerful properties. Each essential oil has its own unique makeup, smell, and healing possibilities. Just because we now have chemical ways to treat conditions faster does not mean that these methods cannot work alongside those methods. We do not recommend ever using essential oils to completely replace medical advice or treatment.

They are intended to be used as a complementary therapy and also to improve general quality of life.

Each essential oil contains different compounds with varied healing and therapeutic benefits. The following are some of the most commonly-used essential oils and the ways in which they can be used.

Frankincense

Frankincense is known as the king of essential oils and is known for providing many health benefits. It has extensive anti-inflammatory properties and it is a good all-rounder by supporting and soothing the mind and body.

- Use frankincense oil in your daily meditation and yoga routine.
- Add frankincense to your skin moisturizer to reduce blemishes and to rejuvenate your skin.
- If you are feeling low try rubbing a few drops of frankincense oil into the soles of your feet to support you.
- Mix three drops of frankincense with a carrier oil and rub right into painful joints.

- Take two drops of 100 percent pure organic therapeutic grade internally to promote healthy cellular function.

Lavender

As one of the most popular essential oils in the world, lavender is well known for its relaxation and calming benefits. Lavender supports good quality of sleep. It is versatile and gentle and a great essential oil to have on hand at all times.

- If you are having trouble sleeping, place a few drops on your pillows or bedding or apply lavender oil to the soles of your feet.
- Add lavender oil to any hair product or conditioner. It keeps the scalp looking clean and healthy.
- Add a drop of lavender oil to your bath water for instant relaxation.
- When you start to feel tension building in your body, apply lavender oil directly on to your temples and back of your neck.

- For an instant solution for all those unwanted smells, combine lavender oil and water in a spray bottle.

Lemon

Lemon essential oil has many benefits for health and a fresh, clean citrus smell which is uplifting for the mind and body. Use this lemon essential oil daily to cleanse your body and physical environment.

- Add lemon essential oil to your drinking water for a delicious taste and to support natural cleansing of the body.
- Add four drops of lemon essential oil to your diffuser if you are struggling to wake up in the morning, and you'll find yourself invigorated and ready to take on the day.
- For a natural cleaner that breaks down grease use: a half cup of water, 1 1/2 cup white vinegar, and 8 drops of lemon oil.
- Add a few drops of lemon oil to your extra virgin olive oil for a cheaper version of infused olive oil than the store-bought, ready-made version.

- To help fight off seasonal allergies, take two drops each of lemon, lavender, and peppermint oils.

Peppermint

There are very few body, health, or mind issues that peppermint oil isn't helpful in relieving. This cooling oil has a calming effect on the body as well as your digestive system.

- Instead of your afternoon cup of coffee for a lift, use a drop of peppermint oil massaged into your temples for an immediate energy boost.

- Three drops of peppermint oil helps to ease nausea when applied to a cold compress.

- Freshen your breath with one drop of peppermint oil in your mouth.

- Before a meal, add a drop of peppermint oil to a glass of water and drink it in order to reduce bloating, gas, and indigestion.

- For a quick pick me up when your energy levels are lagging, apply a few drops of peppermint oil to your hands and inhale deeply.

Ylang Ylang

This calming oil supports your nervous system, helps to reduce tension and anxiety and provides antioxidant support.

- Rub two drops into the back of your neck to relieve tension and stress.

- Rub two drops into the skin over your heart for emotional support.

- When placed in a diffuser, this sweet floral scent is thought to raise your spirits and support you emotionally.

- Naturally stimulate your libido by adding a ylang ylang to your pillows and bed sheets.

- Massaging ylang ylang into your abdomen can provide instant relief from PMS cramps and symptoms.

Essential Oils Specifically for Menopausal Symptoms

Some of the symptoms of menopause can be disruptive in our daily activities. There are homeopathic ways to help you cope despite how uncomfortable these conditions can become. Essential oils may help lessen the severity of some of the symptoms you are experiencing. If prescribed medications are not the way that you want to go, there are alternative options. Some essential oils have been shown to have impacts on symptoms when applied to various parts of the body. Essential oils come from many different plants and can often be found in their original from. You can also purchase essential oils in forms that are ready to apply like creams and oils. With their main use being in aromatherapy, these oils are meant to be inhaled (directly or through a diffuser) or mixed with a carrier oil and applied to the skin.

These five essential oils may help relieve your symptoms:

Clary sage

Hot flashes may be naturally reduced by rubbing three drops of diluted clary sage oil all over your feet or into the skin on the back of your neck. Add a few drops to a tissue, for faster relief, and inhale and exhale gently and evenly, so that the oil enters your body through your nostrils. This breathing process combined with the clary sage oil can produce antidepressant-like effects. Women in menopause have an increased risk for osteoporosis due to a decline in estrogen and during this time, bone breakdown can overtake bone growth. Clary sage is thought to help slow the development of osteoporosis.

Peppermint oil

Peppermint oil may also reduce the discomfort from hot flashes. Dot the oil onto a tissue and slowly breathe in and out while holding it near your nose. It is not uncommon to experience menstrual cramping (dysmenorrhea) during perimenopause. These cramps may even continue after menstruation has ceased completely. This may be a sign of an underlying medical condition. Consult your doctor if you are not menstruating any longer but still experiencing persistent cramping. Peppermint oil may help to relieve this cramping.

Lavender

If the skin around your perineum feels strange, painful or uncomfortable, lavender can help to soothe this discomfort and balance out your hormones. Place a cold cloth enriched with one drop of diluted lavender oil on the area. Only use the cloth for 30 minutes at the most. If there is a stinging sensation, remove the cloth and rinse the skin well with water. During menopause, sleep-related problems such as insomnia are common even if you don't have a history of experiencing such issues. Lavender essential oil can be very helpful in promoting good quality of sleep by relaxing you.

Geranium

As an essential oil, geranium has been found to help menopausal women manage hormonal changes. Drop one or two drops onto a tissue and inhale deeply for immediate stress relief. In your bath water, geranium essential oil is helpful for dry skin. Geranium has antidepressant and antianxiety effects.

Basil

Consider adding basil aromatherapy to your daily regimen to increase your estrogen levels and help improve your mood. Basil can help to relieve hot flashes when applied to the soles of your feet or rubbed into the skin at the back of your neck in a diluted form.

Citrus

Citrus essential oil aromatherapy has many benefits for women who are experiencing menopausal side effects including reducing physical symptoms and increasing libido. It also helps to decrease systolic blood pressure and stabilize pulse rate and estrogen levels. Citrus essential oils also have anti-inflammatory properties for aches and pains. Citrus oils can make your skin photosensitive so avoid direct sunlight if applying diluted citrus oils directly to your skin.

There are some risk factors to consider when using essential oils. Speak you're your doctor before using essential oils for relief of menopausal symptoms as they will be able to tell you if the oils will have any contraindications with medications you may be taking. Also seek medical advice first if you have any known allergies, as some oils may contain potentially allergy-inducing components.

Before using essential oils ensure that you are clear on the instructions ahead of time. Applying undiluted essential oils directly to the skin or ingesting them if they are not food grade can be harmful. Before using essential oils directly on your skin, they should be diluted with a carrier oil. Some examples of popular carrier oils are olive oil and coconut oil. You will also be able to purchase carrier oils wherever you are buying your essential oil products. In order to dilute your essential oil, combine one ounce of the carrier oil with 12 drops of the essential oil of your choice and mix thoroughly.

Perform a patch test, by applying the oil to a small area of skin on the inside of your arm, before doing a full application onto your skin to test for reactions. Wait 24 hours to see if your skin experiences any inflammation or irritation. If you are using an oil in a spray, make sure you're in an area with proper ventilation (Gordon, 2016).

Meditation for Menopausal Symptoms

Meditation does not need to be carried out in a very specific place or in any particular way to be useful. The key behind meditation is focusing on what is happening in the here and now and the best way to do that is by focusing on your breath. Your breath is the lifeforce of your body. It carries oxygen to your organs and helps to rid your body of harmful carbon dioxide. If all you do to begin with, is focus on your breath, you are already meditating.

Sometimes visualizations help us to really maintain focus. When you breathe, picture your breath as a white stream of light that enters your body with a healing purpose. Picture as it fills your lungs and your bloodstream transports little particles of that white light throughout your body until your entire system is glowing white. Then on your outbreath, picture all of the toxins and negative energy that is inside your body being picked up by the stream of light and exiting the body. It is very important to focus as much on your out breath as your in breath. A common mistake when focusing on breath and meditating is to think that the in breath is more important. By doing this you can overload your body with carbon dioxide because you need a good, strong, and extended out breath to push all of the carbon dioxide out. Your out breath can actually be a few seconds longer than your in breath.

When we become anxious, one of the first things that changes is our heart rate and breathing. If we can learn to control our breathing, we can convince our body that our anxiety has moved on and put ourselves back into a physical condition that is relaxed. This also ensures that all of our organs are getting the oxygen they need to function properly. This is especially important for our brains and if you have ever done something that is completely out of character when you are very anxious, it is likely due to a lack of oxygen. If you can get a good supply of oxygen to your brain all of your other faculties will be far easier to manage and you will make better, more reasonable decisions. This helps us, not just to deal with our menopausal symptoms but also when we are fasting. By meditating ourselves into a mindful space we can acknowledge and move on from hunger without giving in to it or allowing it to cause us distress. Meditation can really help us in many areas of our life and there is no magical component to it. All we are doing is refusing to live in the moments we can't control (the past and the future) and instead, we are choosing to only concern ourselves with the present. The entire root of anxiety, of course, is unreasonable stress about things we cannot control. If we acknowledge that we cannot stop our bodies from going into menopause but we do have control over how we deal with it, we are far more likely to be in a calmer state.

There is significant research available to suggest that maintaining a mindful state can help to improve psychological health. The ability of a person to focus on the present moment is the essence of the word 'mindfulness.' Our minds wander very often into the past and the future and this causes stress and anxiety as we are focusing on things that we cannot control rather than on what we can control. When practicing mindfulness, we seek to observe the thoughts that come into our head without judging them; we become better acquainted with ourselves, and we learn to appreciate the present.

A study by Mayo Clinic published in *Climacteric: The Journal of the International Menopause Society,* indicates that mindfulness may help women to experience fewer menopausal symptoms. In this study, it was found that menopausal women with higher mindfulness scores experienced fewer menopausal symptoms. The study consisted of 1,700 women between 40 and 65 years of age and the Mayo Clinic's Women's Health Clinic in Rochester cared for them between January 1, 2015, and December 31, 2016 (Townley, 2019).

Participants completed questionnaires in order to rate their symptoms, how much stress they felt that they were experiencing and how severe they felt that their symptoms were.

Women with higher mindfulness scores experienced fewer symptoms but the impact of mindfulness seemed to be different for the various symptoms. It should also be considered that certain symptoms will be focused on more by certain women. Women who are naturally 'cold-blooded' (don't feel the cold easily) will not necessarily find hot flashes to be as disturbing as women who naturally feel heat excessively.

It is also believed that the reason why mindfulness has different impacts on certain symptoms is that they have more to do with an individual participant's personality. Mindfulness did have a good effect on scores for depression, irritability, and anxiety in middle-aged menopausal women. A woman living with depression and anxiety as a norm, for instance, would likely not even consider those as symptoms of menopause and they would therefore rank far lower on the concern scale than hot flashes perhaps. A woman who has always slept well throughout her life and relies on her eight hours of quality sleep will find the insomnia that sometimes comes from menopause as very difficult to deal with. Our experiences are all very individual and personal.

The goal during mindful moments is to observe the mind's activity while simultaneously being kind to oneself and to create a pause in the mind. It is also intended to help one to observe one's own thoughts and emotions without judgement. The calm that results from this reduces stress and anxiety levels. Mindfulness could become a great tool to help women experiencing menopause who are living with anxiety and depression, according to the data gleaned from the study. It certainly cannot hurt to practice this ancient method of focusing one's thoughts and it will definitely have positive knock-on effects in other areas of life. More research is needed to confirm the effectiveness of this method. That said, because we know that mindfulness is beneficial to psychological health in general, this should certainly be seen as a helpful additional treatment for menopausal symptoms (Townley, 2019).

A study from the University of Pennsylvania found that meditating for just 12 minutes a day improved the moods and even increased the working memory of Marines during deployment. Although we aren't going to war, it does sometimes feel like our body is waging war on itself during menopause. Stress caused by menopause can contribute to memory loss, weight gain, osteoporosis, and even sagging skin. The heart secretes a hormone called atrial natriuretic peptide, which plays a role in the release cortisol which is one of the stress hormones. With every time the heart beats, pressure waves are sent through the arteries. When that pressure reaches the brain, the brain's electrical activity changes. By considering this, it can be determined that your heart can help control how your body responds to stress.

The electromagnetic field around the heart is the most powerful in the body. It is 5,000 times stronger than the electromagnetic field produced by the brain. The electromagnetic field around the heart permeates every cell in our body and can be measured eight feet away from your body. It is quite literally true that people near you can be impacted by the energy of your heart. Meditating therefore doesn't just relax you, it also slows down our heart. When we meditate the interval between each beat of our heart changes and becomes less irregular. The interval between each beat is called the Heart Rate Variability and people with smoother Heart Rate Variability live longer.

You may think that you just don't have time for meditation but when you understand the concept it becomes clear that meditation is not a time-consuming activity. You also don't have to be in any specific place to do it. Meditation revolves around focusing on your breath and that is one of the things that makes it so easy to do. The following are some suggestions on how to incorporate meditation into your daily life in the most surprising places:

Meditate while on the road: Sit up straight and focus your mind on how your body is pressing against the car seat. This is called grounding. Grounding helps you to connect to something immovable when you are in a state of anxiety. If you are connected to something with a solid state then even if your emotions are in flux, you have something to anchor you. Focus on listening to the sounds around you. Listen to how your wheels sound on the road, how your car's engine purrs and even the hooting and sounds of the cars around you. Then focus on each of your other senses for a minute. Focus on each one individually and then allow yourself to tune into them all at the same time. As you are doing this, recognize how all of these components of your environment are not stressful to you but, rather, they all play a role in your present moment and how you fit into that present moment.

Meditate during your lunch break: This is an excellent meditation to use during your eating window to really acknowledge what you are taking into your body. It helps to make you feel less hungry and encourages gratitude for the food you are eating. Focus on each element of your lunch individually. Before you eat it, look at your lunch, take in the colors and the way all of the elements of your meal fit together. Enjoy the aroma of your food. What does it remind you of? When you take your first bite, savor the texture and the way the food feels in your mouth. Chew slowly and deliberately, picturing yourself doing the work to break down your meal so that you are sending digestible nutrients into your system. Focus on each and every bite. All too often we wolf down our food and feel bloated and ill afterwards. By practicing this lunchtime meditation, we can avoid binging and really enjoy our food. Plus, lunch will actually be an enjoyable experience rather than something you rush through so that you can get back to work.

Meditation while in bed: Meditating just before you go to sleep is a great way to relax and prepare your mind for sleep. You can also use this meditation to relax all of your muscles so that you don't go to sleep with tension and experience disturbed sleep. As you lay in bed close your eyes and focus on your breathing. Then start to focus on each of your body parts starting at your toes. Flex your toe muscles and then relax. Then focus on your feet, also flexing and relaxing. Work your way all the way up your body to the top of your head, all the while breathing deeply in and out.

Conclusion

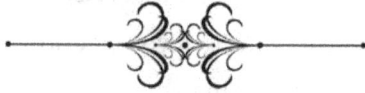

Moving across the crest of 50 can be an anxiety-ridden time for women. The horror stories that we are told about the difficulties of menopause make us wish that we could freeze time and just stay exactly where we are. The truth, though, is that, just like we survived puberty, pregnancy, and every other major change that living in a female body brings, menopause is equally survivable. It impacts every woman differently, simply because each woman's hormonal balance is different, and past experiences with hormonal changes are not really a good way to judge what your menopause will be like. You also cannot compare your experience to your mother's, friend's or sister's experiences of menopause. It's essentially a mountain that we have to climb ourselves and we can't use anyone else's map to guide us. Despite the difficulties that might await us, turning 50 is actually a really exciting time. Your life becomes more focused on your happiness as you watch your family grow and start to focus on themselves. This is your time and you would be remiss not to use it to your full benefit. Making the best of this time will take a little bit of planning and learning but, by completing this book, you have already paved a large part of the path.

Menopause does not have to be something that you suffer through. All of the side effects and symptoms of menopause are treatable and manageable. It may take some lifestyle changes but those small changes will absolutely be worth it. While many medications and procedures exist to treat some of the symptoms of menopause and aging, nothing will ever beat a strong foundation of good nutrition and physical activity. This has to be your starting point, even in your intermittent fasting journey.

In *My Lovely Choice*, we have taken a deep dive into the concept of intermittent fasting. We've explained fasting's ancient origins as well as the science behind what happens in your body when you fast. With all of the fad diets popping up lately, it is refreshing to see a regime that does not simply make claims without proof. For every benefit that fasting claims to produce, there is research and a valid explanation behind how this happens in the body. Truly understanding your body's own processes is the key to sustained health. Sure, you can drive a car without understanding how the engine works, but at the very least if you don't know what fuel to put in, when to check your oil, and when to service your car, you are going to end up with a broken vehicle! The same concept works for your body, regardless of what regimen, eating plan, or diet you are trying. Don't ever try a plan simply because an article or book says it is good for you. It is absolutely imperative that you understand how the benefits are supposed to occur within your body. Not only does this empower you as a woman and a human being but it ensures that you can recognize truly beneficial routines compared to ones that are going to waste your time and very possibly damage your health. If you are considering a route other than fasting and there is not a very decent amount of information, research, and data available on the approach, think twice before trying it. As we age, our bodies heal slower and any damage you do to your body now could be irreversible.

Thankfully, intermittent fasting has centuries of social proof and decades of scientific research behind it. As it only works with your body's existing processes, you are not introducing any foreign activities or substances into your body. The intermittent fasting recommendation of maintaining a healthy whole food diet also makes it far easier to stick to than plans that insist on special food items. With intermittent fasting, you can stick to your usual way of eating as long as it supports nutritional balance and the macronutrients that your body needs. The flexibility of fasting in terms of time periods is also highly beneficial as it means that you can shape fasting around your life and not the other way around. You don't have to make embarrassing excuses as to why you can't join friends for dinner or sit nibbling on a salad while everyone else is enjoying pizza. It is often the inflexibility of eating plans and diets that cause people to fail because we are all human and sometimes life just doesn't bend to our will.

Just 10 years ago, our biggest health issue in the world was the fact that so many people across the world did not have access to proper nutrition. Today, our focus is the very opposite problem, the world is becoming increasingly obese. Overnutrition has become our new plague and is the leading cause of death in the risk factors for chronic disease that it creates. Even if you have never suffered from excessive weight gain in your life, the hormonal changes that inevitably happen in menopause can cause you to gain weight, especially around your belly area. This can be avoided, though, by starting to practice intermittent fasting and making healthier choices about what you eat. It's not necessary to suddenly become a vegetarian (unless you want to) or only eat lettuce leaves all day. You can eat well and you can enjoy your food. Healthy food can be tasty too and you don't have to completely cut out your favorite treat foods either. It is absolutely fine to have the foods that you enjoy, just reduce the frequency with which you eat them and don't eat them just before a fast as your body needs good nutrition during that time.

While weight loss is an important factor in maintaining our health as we age, autophagy is a really beneficial process in so many ways. If you have ever spent huge amounts of money on anything that purports to be 'anti-aging,' you can stop now, because autophagy is free. The process of autophagy when accelerated by fasting can clear up your skin, rejuvenate your organs, rebuild your immune system and help to prevent cancer and degenerative brain diseases.

As a woman over 50, it is vital that you understand the mechanics of what is happening to your body as you enter menopause. This will make the experience far less intimidating and you will feel empowered and in control. You owe it to yourself and your family to embrace the availability of knowledge and make this experience the best that it can be. Knowing what to expect from menopause is perhaps half the battle already won as you can prepare and avoid feeling desperate and lost.

Our mental health needs to be a major focus for us during this time as, even if you have never suffered from depression or anxiety, menopause is a time during which these conditions can develop in many women. Support groups are a great way to air your frustrations and talk to others experiencing the same things as you and, today, these are available on social media as well as in person, so you can have 24-hour support no matter where you are. Yoga, meditation, and practicing mindfulness all help to support your mental health and keep you focused in the moment. Keep a keen eye on your relationships during this time and be careful not to get so wrapped up in your own experiences that you fail to see how you are impacting others. Your family and friends love you and only want the best for you but they may not know how to deal with you if your behavior becomes significantly different. The only way they will know what you need from them in terms of support is if you tell them. This is equally applicable in your intermittent fasting journey as it is in your menopause.

If your family is not planning on fasting with you, make sure that you explain to everyone exactly what you are going to be doing and why you are doing it. Besides you, your family and friends are going to be the greatest beneficiaries of the results of your fasting journey. You will have an improved mood, better health, more energy, and a clearer mind, so really this journey is in their best interests too. Your family and friends do not have to agree with your choice in order to support you and be sure to make this clear to them as well. All you really need from them, is for them not to stand in your way, or purposefully sabotage your efforts for any reason. With that being said, your probability of success will always be in your hands. You are the one who has chosen this journey and only you can make sure that you are successful.

There are many different ways to do intermittent fasting, and there is no single plan that will work for everyone. Individuals will experience the best outcomes if they try out the various methods to see what suits their lifestyle and preferences. Regardless of the type of fasting, fasting for extended periods when the body is not ready can be tricky. Remember, fasting may not be suitable for everyone. If a person is prone to disordered eating, these approaches may aggravate their unhealthy relationship with food. People with health conditions, including diabetes, should speak to a doctor before attempting any form of fasting. For the best results, it is essential to eat a healthy and balanced diet on non-fasting days. If necessary, a person can seek professional help to personalize an intermittent fasting plan and avoid pitfalls.

People have practiced fasting for thousands of years, but its safety depends more on who is doing the fasting than the style of fasting itself. People who have malabsorption, are at risk of low blood sugar, or have other medical conditions should seek the counsel of their healthcare provider. While most people can practice many fasting styles safely, extreme types of intermittent fasting, can lead to inadequate intake of nutrients such as fiber, vitamins, and minerals. Therefore, people should approach this style of fasting with caution.

Many people will have different opinions about fasting and that is just fine. We need to base our decisions on facts and research. We encourage you to go beyond this resource and look into other aspects of fasting so that you really feel comfortable about the decision you are making. When you start to experience the benefits of fasting, it is helpful to your own journey to share that information with others and ensure that you are giving your friends, sister and daughters the same gift of being able to manage their own journey through life. It has taken us some to come back to the idea of fasting as a society and while it is not yet a universal lifestyle, more and more people including doctors and other medical practitioners are starting to acknowledge the benefits that fasting brings to our lives. Although we have focused on the role of fasting and autophagy in women's lives in this book, it certainly has just as much benefit for men over the age of 50. Although they don't experience as many issues with hormones, men do also have very particular health concerns as they age which can be addressed by fasting. Men actually tend to adopt a fasting lifestyle far easier than they would a calorie restriction type diet as it is simple and easy to follow. Men also don't need to have as many considerations around the delicate balance of hormones as it relates to fasting so they can fast more intensely and see quicker results. If you have started to experience benefits in your life from starting an intermittent fasting lifestyle, we highly recommend suggesting it to your partner, brother, or father as a way to improve their health and ensure that you have them with you for longer.

A few things that make it tougher to lose weight after age 50 include lower metabolism, achy joints, reduced muscle mass, and even sleep issues. At the same time, losing dangerous belly fat, can significantly reduce your risk for such serious health issues as diabetes, heart attacks, and cancer. As you age, of course, the risk for developing many diseases increases. In some cases, intermittent fasting for women over 50 could serve as a virtual fountain of youth when it comes to weight loss and minimizing the chance of developing typically age-related illnesses. Getting rid of additional weight is also a great boon to your emotional and mental health. When you feel better about yourself, you are able to achieve more and it becomes a circle of success. Our day-to-day lives can be difficult enough to manage without the added stress of poor health, so it stands to reason that we would take hold of the tools that we have been given to naturally improve our health. The speed with which you will see results is always going to depend on the base off of which you are starting. Some people naturally have several health issues that they need to work on, and if you are one such person, you will need to choose which to focus on first. The best bet is always to address your weight first as well as your nutrition as those two places are often where disease and chronic conditions start. Once you have managed to rid yourself of the extra weight, you can reassess and see where you are at that point, from a health perspective, and work from there.

Intermittent fasting is not a cure-all method for every ailment and there are people for whom intermittent fasting doesn't work in the way it does for most others. You will never know which group you fall into, though, unless you try it. You may be able to fast with absolutely no side effects or you may need to very carefully craft your eating and fasting window to fit into a schedule that works for you. The ultimate goal, no matter how you decide to do it, is to increase the amount of time that your body spends in a fasted state. If you are not fasting at all and you are able to fast for only one day a week, that is still progress. You have spent 50 years living in your body and you can spend another 50 repairing it if you need to, but you have to take that first step otherwise the journey will never start.

If you have been told that, as you enter your 50s it's time to slow down and not try anything new so that you can retain your energy to 'suffer' through your menopause, it's time for you to prove them wrong. As much as it may feel as though these things are happening to you and your body is turning against you, that is not the case at all. Just as puberty prepared you for a new stage in your life, so does menopause, and honestly, it is easily the most enjoyable stage as it is all about what makes you happy and healthy. Aging does not have to mean you become frail, forgetful, and lose your independence. You are entirely in control of what this stage of your life holds for you. If you treat your body like a dumping ground, it will behave like one. Even if you have never been one to care for your body in the past, it is not too late to change the paradigm. Your body can heal itself if you give it the opportunity and the right tools to do so, and intermittent fasting is the way to achieve that. Take it one day at a time and focus only on the task at hand and you will soon reap the benefits. Please be kind enough to help share the knowledge that you have gleaned from reading My Lovely Choice by writing a review on Amazon, **or subscribe to the newsletter located at Athenapublications.com to be updated on my new editions.** I look forward to hearing about the topics and tips you enjoyed most as well as your intermittent fasting successes. Let's do this!

References

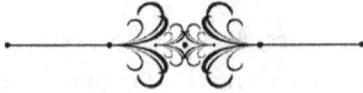

5 Proven Benefits of Intermittent Fasting for People Over 50--and How to Do It. (n.d.). Thrive Naturals. Retrieved April 5, 2020, from https://www.thrivenaturals.com/5-Proven-Benefits-of-Intermittent-Fasting-for-People-Over-50and-How-to-Do-It.html#

6 Intermittent Fasting Mistakes to Avoid | Nutrition | MyFitnessPal. (2019, April 25). Under Armour. https://blog.myfitnesspal.com/6-intermittent-fasting-mistakes-to-avoid/

7 Useful Reminders for Every Woman Going Through Menopause. (n.d.). Healthline. Retrieved April 5, 2020, from https://www.healthline.com/health/menopause/reminders-for-symptoms#1

7 ways to do intermittent fasting: Best methods and quick tips. (n.d.). Www.Medicalnewstoday.Com. https://www.medicalnewstoday.com/articles/322293

Antunes, F., Erustes, A., Costa, A., Nascimento, A., Bincoletto, C., Ureshino, R., Pereira, G., & Smaili, S. (2018). Autophagy and intermittent fasting: the connection for cancer therapy? Clinics, 73(Suppl 1). https://doi.org/10.6061/clinics/2018/e814s

Brazier, Y. (2017, April 26). The raw food diet: Should I try it? Medicalnewstoday.Com; Medical News Today. https://www.medicalnewstoday.com/articles/7381#Video-How-to-start-a-raw-food-diet

English, N. (2016, July 4). Autophagy: The Real Way to Cleanse Your Body. Greatist; Healthline Media. https://greatist.com/live/autophagy-fasting-exercise

Essential Oils for Everyday Living: Fasting Support ⋆ The Wellness Universe Blog. (2019, June 26). The Wellness Universe Blog. https://blog.thewellnessuniverse.com/essential-oils-for-everyday-living-fasting-support/

Fasting. (2019). In Encyclopædia Britannica. https://www.britannica.com/topic/fasting#ref330445

Foods That Can Help Keep Your Hormones Balanced. (n.d.). Bustle. Retrieved April 7, 2020, from https://www.bustle.com/p/10-foods-that-can-help-balance-your-hormones-naturally-3601864

hollowc2. (2019, April 30). Intermittent Fasting: 4 Different Types Explained. Health Essentials from Cleveland Clinic; Health Essentials from Cleveland Clinic. https://health.clevelandclinic.org/intermittent-fasting-4-different-types-explained/

How to Lose Menopause Belly Fat - Foods That Beat Hormone Problems. (2015, December 2). Dr Becky Fitness. https://www.drbeckyfitness.com/how-to-lose-menopause-belly-fat-foods-that-beat-hormone-problems/

How to Renew Your Body: Fasting and Autophagy. (2016, October 5). Diet Doctor. https://www.dietdoctor.com/renew-body-fasting-autophagy

https://www.facebook.com/jamesclear, & Clear, J. (2012, December 10). The Beginner's Guide to Intermittent Fasting. James Clear. https://jamesclear.com/the-beginners-guide-to-intermittent-fasting

https://www.facebook.com/jamesclear, & Clear, J. (2012, December 10). The Beginner's Guide to Intermittent Fasting. James Clear. https://jamesclear.com/the-beginners-guide-to-intermittent-fasting

Intermittent Fasting 101 — The Ultimate Beginner's Guide. (n.d.). Healthline. https://www.healthline.com/nutrition/intermittent-fasting-guide#effects

Intermittent Fasting Food List: What to Eat and Avoid. (2019, September 19). DoFasting. https://dofasting.com/blog/intermittent-fasting-food-list/

Intermittent Fasting for Women Over 50 - Good or Bad? (2017, November 6). Dr Becky Fitness. https://www.drbeckyfitness.com/intermittent-fasting-for-women-over-50/

Intermittent Fasting Morning Workouts for Optimal Fat Loss. (2019, February 18). Yoga Rove. https://yogarove.com/intermittent-fasting-morning-workout/

Is Intermittent Fasting Destroying Your Hormone Balance? (2019, July 26). HealthcoachFX. https://www.healthcoachfx.com/intermittent-fasting-women-hormone-balance/

Jeanie Lerche Davis. (2007, March 23). Get-Fit Advice for Women Over 50. WebMD; WebMD. **https://www.webmd.com/women/guide/women-over-50-fitness-tips**

Jerisha Parker Gordon. (2016, April 15). Can Essential Oils Provide Menopause Relief? Healthline; Healthline Media. https://www.healthline.com/health/menopause/essential-oils-for-menopause#outlook

Kegel exercises - self-care: MedlinePlus Medical Encyclopedia. (n.d.). Medlineplus.Gov. https://medlineplus.gov/ency/patientinstructions/000141.htm

Kresser, C. (2019, March 25). Intermittent Fasting: The Science Behind the Trend. Chris Kresser; chriskresser.com. https://chriskresser.com/intermittent-fasting-the-science-behind-the-trend/

Lindberg, S. (2018, October 26). How to Exercise Safely During Intermittent Fasting. Healthline; Healthline Media. https://www.healthline.com/health/how-to-exercise-safely-intermittent-fasting#1

Longo, V. D., & Mattson, M. P. (2014). Fasting: Molecular Mechanisms and Clinical Applications. Cell Metabolism, 19(2), 181–192. **https://doi.org/10.1016/j.cmet.2013.12.00**8

Lowery, M. (n.d.). Common Mistakes When It Comes To Intermittent Fasting. Vegan News, Plant Based Living, Food, Health & More. Retrieved April 6, 2020, from https://www.plantbasednews.org/lifestyle/common-mistakes-intermittent-fasting

Low Estrogen Symptoms: Identification, Treatment, and More. (n.d.). Healthline. https://www.healthline.com/health/womens-health/low-estrogen-symptoms

Mangan, P. D. (2019, May 24). The Sweet Spot for Intermittent Fasting. Medium. **https://medium.com/better-humans/the-sweet-spot-for-intermittent-fasting-9aae12a2158c**

Mann, D., Feb. 14, Msu., & 2019. (n.d.). 50 Health Secrets Every Woman Over 50 Should Know. The Healthy. Retrieved April 6, 2020, from https://www.thehealthy.com/aging/healthy-aging/health-secrets-women-over-50/

Meditation May Cool Hot Flashes. (n.d.). WebMD. Retrieved April 5, 2020, from https://www.webmd.com/menopause/news/20060913/meditation-may-cool-hot-flashes

Must-Do Strength Training Moves for Women Over 50. (n.d.). Verywell Fit. Retrieved April 7, 2020, from https://www.verywellfit.com/must-do-strength-training-women-over-50-3498202

Sexperts & Personal Trainers Alike Say These 5 Workouts Can Seriously Boost Your Libido. (n.d.). Elite Daily. Retrieved April 7, 2020, from https://www.elitedaily.com/p/5-exercises-that-can-boost-your-libido-for-a-better-sex-life-according-to-experts-16807985

The 6 biggest health mistakes women make in their 50s. (n.d.). TODAY.Com. Retrieved April 5, 2020, from https://www.today.com/health/six-biggest-health-mistakes-women-make-their-50s-t48466

(2020). Valterlongo.Com. https://valterlongo.com/cardiovascular-diseases/

What You Need to Know About Menopause. (n.d.). Healthline. https://www.healthline.com/health/menopause#symptoms

www.ingramcontent.com/pod-product-compliance
Lightning Source LLC
Chambersburg PA
CBHW060839280326
41934CB00007B/853